The Bridge Between
A&P and Pathophysiology

Patricia S. Bowne
Biology Department
Alverno College

Every book about the human body is incomplete and contains errors, because we don't know the full truth about the body.
Every condensed book is an inaccurate oversimplification.
I have tried to make this book as accurate as possible, while keeping it oversimplified.
Egregious errors in describing accepted principles of Anatomy and Physiology or Pathophysiology as of 2019 are my fault, and I will appreciate being told about them.
Inaccuracies arising from newer discoveries are to be expected, but must be blamed on the human body or on science in general.

What Pathophysiology students say:

"The Bridge helped me to be successful in pathophysiology by giving me a condensed review of Anatomy and Physiology... It helped me to save a lot of time on review and contributed a great deal to my understanding of pathophysiology. I especially found The Bridge very helpful because Pat used very simple, easy to understand language"

"It was informative for me and I actually understood the material. It was written to where anyone could follow."

"I really liked the setup of this chapter because it was in short paragraphs and bullet points. This makes the material seem more attainable and organized as opposed to a typical textbook. I also liked that there was an explanation of "what goes wrong". I feel a lot of textbooks emphasize how things should work, but don't explain what the repercussions would be if they don't."

"The set up of two columns with the normal kidney physiology on one side and the what if it goes wrong on the other was a very accessible way to learn about the kidney diseases. It offers quick information in a very clear way."

"I love the short paragraph format of this. It is super helpful to make sure I understand the basics of each system. I specifically liked the "Apply It" exercise in the liver overview because it allows for a more clinical perspective."

"The test yourself section helped me solidify the review and test my ability to recall important vocabulary."

"I liked how it broke down in sections describing the functions of the different parts of the kidneys and what happens if something wrong were to happen with that particular section of the kidney. It was easy to read and comprehend and I like how it walked through flow of the filtration process from beginning to end."

"I absolutely enjoyed the information and the read about each step. This paper would have been a huge help in A & P 202 when we were going over the renal functions; I found it easy to understand."

What instructors say:

"… an incredibly useful tool for my students in pathophysiology. I loved the pacing: quick review followed by a short quiz and then application questions. Also, it was great to have the key available to students to check their own answers (I didn't have to fill in and create the keys… which was wonderful as well!). Students thought these were very helpful in class. … it would be useful for anyone teaching pathophysiology... definitely an unfilled niche."

Susan E. Dentel , Washtenaw Community College

Introduction

THIS IS NOT AN A&P TEXTBOOK.

IT IS NOT A PATHOPHYSIOLOGY TEXTBOOK.

SO WHAT IS IT?

This is a review booklet for people who took A&P and are going to take Pathophysiology. And are nervous.

Perhaps you took your A&P years ago, and aren't sure you know the basics you need for Pathophysiology. Perhaps you're not sure you remember last semester's A&P well enough to apply it to sick people. This book tries to boil the basics down to 1-2 pages per system, with a test-yourself summary sheet for each.

In A&P, you learned the body systems and how they work, but you didn't learn much about what happens when they don't work – except that you did, without focusing on it. If you know the parts of a system, you know the parts that can go wrong. If you know just what each step does, you can figure out what will happen when the step doesn't do its job. That's Pathophysiology, and a big part of it is just thinking a little differently – looking at the steps of a pathway with a 'what if --?' attitude instead of a 'this is what happens' attitude.

The second goal of this book is to give you practice in the 'what if --?' approach. This book will not tell you about any specific diseases; it will review the steps of the normal pathways and what happens if they don't work. When you learn actual diseases in your Pathophysiology class, you should recognize the steps with which they interfere, and be able to 'what if --?' your way to understanding, rather than memorizing, the consequences for your patient.

I wrote this for my own Pathophysiology students. I know it's working when they ask me 'what if?' questions in class. I hope it helps you to ask the same questions, and figure out the same kinds of answers – because someday you will probably be taking care of me.

The information used in these activities is consistent with Grossman, Sheila C., and Carol Mattson Porth (2014) Porth's *Pathophysiology* (9th edition) Wolters Kluwer, so far as I can manage. I have provided sources for any information that is not in Porth's text.

HORMONES are in capital letters throughout, as are other terms I want to draw your attention to.

Contents

The Bridge Between – Stress Response and Stress

Normal Stress Response function	What if it Goes Wrong?
Stress, pain, fear, and low blood pressure activate a set of emergency responses known as the Generalized Stress Response. This response includes: Sympathetic Nervous System activation (SNS) Renin-ANGIOTENSIN-ALDOSTERONE System (RAAS) CORTISOL release ANTIDIURETIC HORMONE release (ADH)	If you couldn't use the generalized stress response, you could find yourself unable to stay alive in conditions of severe stress, like low blood pressure. Because the consequences can be so severe, it's no wonder there are so many systems that can help with this response!
Sympathetic Nervous System Activation	
Sympathetic nerves release norepinephrine (noradrenaline) to stimulate end organs to help you survive an emergency. One of the first end organs stimulated is the adrenal medulla, which releases EPINEPHRINE (ADRENALIN) into the blood. This means the rest of your organs can get sympathetic stimulus from both nerves and the blood.	Without the adrenal medulla, your sympathetic response might be weakened. If the adrenal medulla were overactive, you could have an extreme sympathetic response at a time when it wasn't needed. (Fung, Viveros, &O'Connor, 2008)
Norepinephrine and EPINEPHRINE attach to alpha-1 receptors on arteriolar smooth muscle cells. This causes them to constrict, vasoconstricting the arterioles in the skin, guts, and kidneys. This vasoconstriction increases peripheral resistance (PR) to blood flow, raising the blood pressure in your major arteries.	If you lacked norepinephrine or the alpha-1 receptors were blocked, you would not be able to effectively increase PR and raise blood pressure. With too much alpha-1 receptor stimulation, the kidneys, guts, and skin might not get enough blood flow.
Alpha-2 receptors are present in the central nervous system. When stimulated, they decrease SNS activity. They also decrease GI motility and INSULIN secretion (Marieb & Hoehn, 2016), raising your blood glucose to give you quick energy.	Without alpha-2 receptors, your sympathetic system could run out of control.
Beta-1 receptors on the heart make it beat faster and more strongly.	If beta-1 receptors didn't function, the heart rate and strength would not increase.
Beta-2 receptors are in the skeletal muscle's blood vessels and the bronchioles of the lungs. They make these relax, increasing blood flow to the muscles and making it easier to breathe.	If beta-2 receptors didn't work, your bronchioles would not dilate. You would have trouble breathing.

Renin-ANGIOTENSIN-ALDOSTERONE System (RAAS)	
When blood flow to the kidneys decreases, the kidneys activate the Renin-ANGIOTENSIN-ALDOSTERONE system (RAAS) to raise blood pressure	If you couldn't activate this pathway, you would have trouble raising blood pressure. If you activated it too much, you would develop high blood pressure.
The RAAS turns on when special cells in the kidneys called juxtaglomerular cells (or granular cells) sense low blood pressure in the renal arterioles. These cells can also be directly stimulated by the sympathetic system. They release an enzyme, renin, into the blood.	Without renin, you would not be able to increase blood pressure as effectively.
Renin reacts with the protein angiotensinogen in the blood to form ANGIOTENSIN I. When the blood containing ANGIOTENSIN I passes through the lungs, an enzyme called ANGIOTENSIN converting enzyme converts it into ANGIOTENSIN II.	If you didn't have enough angiotensinogen or ANGIOTENSIN converting enzyme, this pathway would not work and you could not raise blood pressure as effectively.
ANGIOTENSIN II helps to increase blood pressure in several ways: - It causes you to feel thirsty and drink water, increasing your blood volume - It vasoconstricts, increasing PR - It causes the proximal tubules of the kidneys to reabsorb more sodium - It causes the adrenal cortex to release the hormone ALDOSTERONE	Without ANGIOTENSIN II, you would not be able to raise blood pressure as effectively. With too much of it, you could develop high blood pressure.
ALDOSTERONE is called a mineralocorticoid because it helps control the levels of Na^+ and K^+ in the blood. It causes the kidneys to activate an ion pump which reabsorbs 3 Na^+ from the urine into the blood, and secretes 2 K^+ from the blood into the urine. Water follows the majority of ions by osmosis – which means it returns to the blood.	If you had too much ALDOSTERONE, you would retain too much Na^+ and water and lose too much K^+ in your urine. If you had too little ALDOSTERONE, you would lose too much Na^+ and water in your urine, and retain too much K^+ in your blood.

CORTISOL release	
When you are stressed, your hypothalamus releases CORTICOTROPIN RELEASING HORMONE (CRH) to your anterior pituitary. The anterior pituitary then releases CORTICOTROPIN or ADRENAL COTRICOTROPHIC HORMONE (ACTH) into the circulation. ACTH causes the adrenal cortex to releaseCORTISOL into the blood. CORTISOL is also called the stress hormone. It makes your cells release stored glucose and break down fat and muscle. Some of these compounds are converted to glucose, raising your blood glucose levels. CORTISOL also strengthens your response to the sympathetic system. It decreases inflammation, immune system function and the creation of fibroblasts, cells involved in skin repair and scar tissue.	With low levels ofCORTISOL, you wouldn't be able to raise blood glucose when your cells needed it to help deal with stress. Your blood pressure might also decrease. With high levels ofCORTISOL, your blood glucose might go too high. With long periods of highCORTISOL, your muscles might become weak as protein breaks down. Fat would move from your arms and legs to your head, neck, and trunk. Your immune system would be suppressed, and your skin might become thin.

ANTIDIURETIC HORMONE release (ADH)	
If your body is dehydrated, the cells in your hypothalamus will secrete ANTIDIURETIC HORMONE (ADH, also called VASOPRESSIN). This hormone makes the nephrons in your kidneys more permeable to water, so water in the urine can move into your blood by osmosis and correct the dehydration.	If you couldn't make ADH, you wouldn't be able to reabsorb water from your urine sufficiently. You'd always be urinating, and would have to keep drinking to avoid dehydration. If you made too much ADH, you'd always be moving water from your urine into your blood, and your blood might become too dilute. Then your cells would swell.

Fung, M. M., Viveros, O. H., & O'Connor, D. T. (2008). Diseases of the adrenal medulla. Acta Physiologica (Oxford, England), 192(2), 325–335. https://doi.org/10.1111/j.1748-1716.2007.01809.x
Marieb, E.H., and K. Hoehn, 2016. Human Anatomy & Physiology, 10th ed. Pearson.

Test yourself! Stress Response and Stress

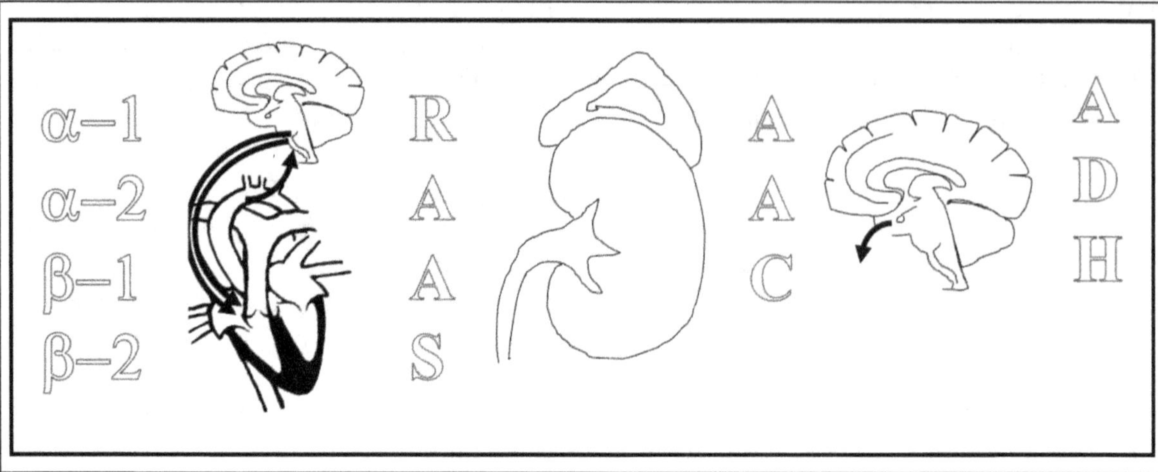

Here's your brain, noticing that you're in trouble.

You might have ______, ______, ______, or ____________.
These problems will make the brain turn on the ________________ nervous system, which will release ____________________ from neurons to the target cells and make the adrenal medulla put ____________________ into the blood.

When these compounds attach to ________ receptors, blood vessels in the ______, ______, and ________ constrict. ________ receptors make the heartbeat faster and stronger. Beta-2 receptors dilate blood vessels in ____________ so you can run away faster, and ____________ bronchioles so you can breathe more easily. And ________ receptors inhibit further release of ________________, so the system doesn't run out of control.

Your kidneys also notice a problem; their blood flow has ____________!

Special cells called ____________________ cells release __________ into the blood. This enzyme converts ________________ into ____________________ and the ____________ ____________ enzyme in the lungs further converts that into ______________.

____________ helps raise your blood pressure by making you __________, by ____________ blood vessels, and by causing the kidneys to ________ ______ ____ ____ ______. It also causes __________ to be secreted from your adrenal ______.
ALDOSTERONE makes the kidneys __________ ______ ___ ______ and ____________ ______ into the urine.

Your adrenal gland is really busy helping with the stress response.

The adrenal __________ is releasing ____________ to help the SNS. The adrenal ____________ is releasing ____________ to help the RAAS. And the adrenal cortex is also releasing ________, the stress hormone that ______ your blood glucose and suppresses your ________ response.

The last part of the generalized stress response is ____________ hormone, which is released from the hypothalamus. This causes your kidneys to reabsorb ______ from your urine into the blood, __________ blood volume.

Apply it! Stress Response and Stress

Mr. O went buffalo hunting, but the buffalo got him instead! His buddies had to drive him back to the nearest town, and he was losing blood all the way. When he arrived at the ER he was pale and his skin was cold; he had a rapid heartbeat and his blood glucose was elevated. Which part(s) of the generalized stress response were causing this? What made them turn on and how were they causing his signs and symptoms?

Though it took them two hours to reach the hospital and he drank a whole bottle of water, Mr. O didn't produce any urine on the way. What prevented him from producing urine? What made him thirsty?

The medical team sprang into action, stopping his bleeding and giving him an IV to replace blood volume. An hour later, he was more comfortable – but he still hadn't produced any urine. The med student said, "That's normal, isn't it?"
"Just barely," said the doctor. "I'm getting worried about it."
What could happen to Mr. O if his stress response stays on for too long?

The Bridge Between – Inflammation and Inflammatory Disorders

Normal Inflammatory function	What if it Goes Wrong?
So, you hurt yourself. The damaged cells will release inflammatory mediators, compounds that start an inflammation. These include prostaglandins, thromboxane A2, and leukotrienes, which are made from arachidonic acid found in the cell membrane.	If you didn't have enough arachidonic acid, you wouldn't be able to make enough of these inflammatory mediators. A diet that decreased arachidonic acid might reduce inflammation (Campos-Staffico *et al.*, 2019).
Prostaglandins and thromboxane A2 are made by the cyclooxygenase pathway. Some prostaglandins cause inflammation; others do other functions, like protecting the stomach lining or increasing blood flow to the kidneys.	Aspirin works by blocking the cyclooxygenase pathway. If you couldn't make prostaglandins, you might have less inflammation. But you also might not be able to protect your stomach lining, and that's why aspirin is hard on the stomach.
Thromboxane A2 promotes platelet function – clotting.	If you didn't make thromboxane A2, you would have decreased platelet plug formation. This is one reason aspirin is often prescribed for people who are at risk of forming blood clots.
It's not just the damaged cells that respond to injury! There are some leukocytes (white blood cells or WBCs) called mast cells living in the tissues. When the tissue is injured, these cells also release inflammatory mediators, including histamine.	If you blocked histamine, you could decrease the development of an inflammation. That's one reason we take antihistamines.
All these inflammatory mediators have an effect on the blood vessels running through the injured tissue. They cause vasodilation and increased permeability – so more blood enters the area, but lots of the fluid and protein leaks out into the tissue. This is called an exudate.	If this effect is too large or widespread, the vasodilation and loss of fluid from the blood could cause blood pressure to drop dangerously low. If too much fluid leaked out into a tissue, the pressure in the tissue might rise far enough to interfere with blood flow. Or the fluid might interfere with the tissue's function – for instance, exudate in the lungs could affect breathing.
Blood vessels also begin to display adhesive proteins on their linings (Granger & Senchenkova, 2010). These provide places for passing white blood cells to catch on to, so they can enter the injured tissue.	If you didn't have these proteins, WBCs might not effectively enter the injured tissues. You would be less able to fight off infections.

These effects on blood vessels are called the VASCULAR RESPONSE. Once the WBCs arrive, the CELLULAR RESPONSE has begun.	The vascular response causes the primary signs of inflammation – heat, redness, swelling, and pain. If it didn't happen, the tissues wouldn't get the blood flow needed to help them repair the injury – or the WBCs they would need to fight off infection.
The first white blood cells that enter the damaged tissue are mostly neutrophils, or polymorphonuclear leukocytes (that means 'many-shaped nuclei). They eat pathogens and damaged tissue, attract more WBCs, and also secrete inflammatory mediators and enzymes that can break down damaged tissue.	If neutrophils kept entering an area, they could start to damage healthy tissue. This is a factor in many chronic wounds or chronic inflammations. If there weren't enough neutrophils, then you would be less able to kill off pathogens and more prone to infection.
WBCs called Monocytes are then attracted to the area. They mature into macrophages (that means 'big eaters') and begin to eat pathogens in the injured tissue. They also secrete many compounds that are involved with both inflammation and healing. Macrophages are a major source of compounds called cytokines, which enter the bloodstream and travel throughout the body. They cause fever, aches and pains, malaise (feeing 'sick'), and increased WBC production, and increase the inflammatory response. This is called the acute-phase response, or systemic inflammation.	Diseases that reduce the number of macrophages could interfere with your ability to fight off diseases and to heal properly. High levels of cytokines could cause dangerously high fevers, and lower the blood pressure by stimulating the vascular response (Tisoncik *et al.*, 2012)

Campos-Staffico, A. M., Costa, A. P. R., Carvalho, L. S. F., Moura, F. A., Santos, S. N., Coelho-Filho, O. R., … Sposito, A. C. (2019). Omega-3 intake is associated with attenuated inflammatory response and cardiac remodeling after myocardial infarction. *Nutrition Journal, 18*. https://doi.org/10.1186/s12937-019-0455-1

Granger, D. N., & Senchenkova, E. (2010). Leukocyte–Endothelial Cell Adhesion. Morgan & Claypool Life Sciences. Retrieved from https://www.ncbi.nlm.nih.gov/books/NBK53380/

Tisoncik, J. R., Korth, M. J., Simmons, C. P., Farrar, J., Martin, T. R., & Katze, M. G. (2012). Into the Eye of the Cytokine Storm. Microbiology and Molecular Biology Reviews : MMBR, 76(1), 16–32. https://doi.org/10.1128/MMBR.05015-11

Test yourself! Inflammation and Inflammatory Disorders

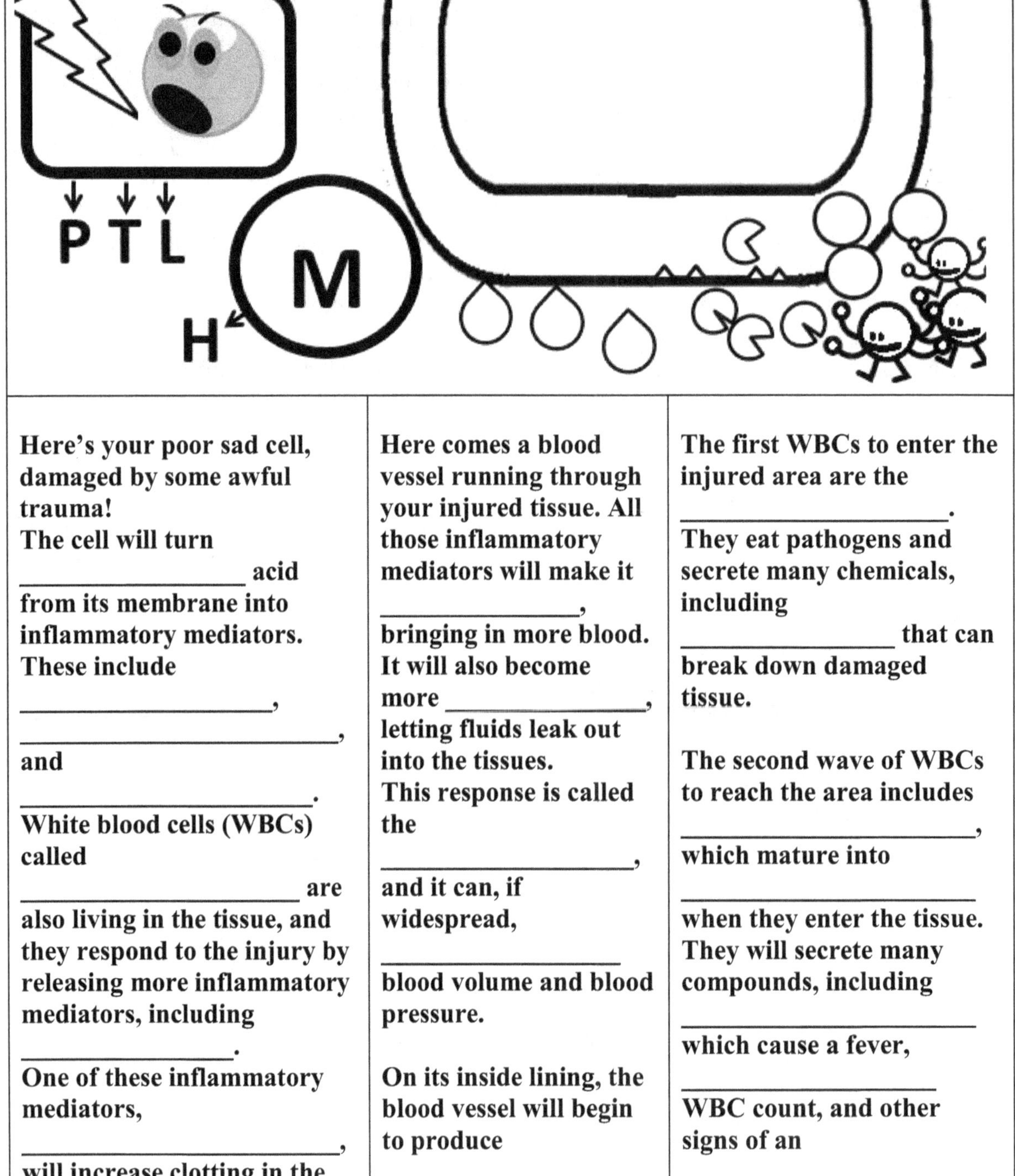

Here's your poor sad cell, damaged by some awful trauma!
The cell will turn

_________________ acid from its membrane into inflammatory mediators. These include

_________________,

_________________,

and

_________________.

White blood cells (WBCs) called

_________________ are also living in the tissue, and they respond to the injury by releasing more inflammatory mediators, including

_________________.

One of these inflammatory mediators,

_________________,

will increase clotting in the injured area.

Here comes a blood vessel running through your injured tissue. All those inflammatory mediators will make it

_________________,

bringing in more blood. It will also become more _________________, letting fluids leak out into the tissues.
This response is called the

_________________,

and it can, if widespread,

____

blood volume and blood pressure.

On its inside lining, the blood vessel will begin to produce

____

proteins to catch passing WBCs.

The first WBCs to enter the injured area are the

_________________.

They eat pathogens and secrete many chemicals, including

_________________ that can break down damaged tissue.

The second wave of WBCs to reach the area includes

_________________,

which mature into

____

when they enter the tissue. They will secrete many compounds, including

____

which cause a fever,

____

WBC count, and other signs of an

____

or _________________ response.

Sad cell from Microsoft clip art, 2013

The Bridge Between – Immune System and Immune Disorders

Normal Adaptive Immunity	What if it Goes Wrong?
Adaptive immunity means immunity against a specific thing. Your body identifies these things by molecules on their surfaces, or ANTIGENS.	If the thing infecting your body had no antigens on its surface, your immune system would not respond to it. If your body reacted to something that wasn't really dangerous as if it were an antigen, it might start an allergic reaction to that substance. If your body reacted to one of your normal proteins as if it were an antigen, you might develop an autoimmune disease and damage your own tissues.
When your tissue is damaged, an inflammatory reaction starts. The inflammatory mediators created in that reaction attract WBC, including MACROPHAGES and DENDRITIC CELLS. Macrophages, dendritic cells and some other WBCs can act as ANTIGEN-PRESENTING CELLS or APCs. These cells collect the antigen from an infected area and present it to the immune cells.	Without APCs, you wouldn't be able to develop immunity against specific pathogens (Bigley, Barge, & Collin, 2016).
The APC eats the antigen and breaks it into little pieces called epitopes. It then puts these on special proteins on its surfaces. These proteins are called MHC-II proteins (mutual histocompatibility complex).	If there weren't any MHC-II proteins, the APCs wouldn't be able to display the epitopes and your immune cells would never see them (Reith & Mach, 2001).
The APC then leaves the damaged tissue and travels up a lymph vessel until it reaches a lymph node.	If the APC couldn't travel up the lymph vessel, it would not be as able to tell the immune system about the infection (Bigley, Barge, & Collin, 2016).
In the lymph node, your immune cells or lymphocytes are waiting. There are two main types: B cells and T cells. T cells are divided into T helper (CD4+) cells, T cytotoxic (CD8+) cells, and T regulatory cells.	If you didn't have lymphocytes, you wouldn't be able to create an adaptive immune response.

B and T cells are individuals – that is, while there are many B cells, each cell may have different cell surface receptors, which can attach to different antigens.	If you didn't happen to have any B or T cells with receptors that fit a particular antigen, you would be unable to begin an immune response against that antigen.
The APC presents (or shows) the antigen to the T helper cells in the lymph node. When it meets a T helper cell with a receptor for that antigen, that T helper cell becomes activated. It begins to divide into T helper 1 (Th1) and T helper 2 (Th2) cells. and to secrete cytokines.	If the APC didn't find a T cell with a receptor that could attach to the antigen, you would not be able to start an adaptive immune response against that antigen.
Th1 cells stimulate T cytotoxic cells that have the same antigen receptors they have, and Th2 cells stimulate B cells that have the same antigen receptors they have. They activate those B cells and T cytotoxic cells.	Without Th1 cells, you would not be able to activate the T cytotoxic cells. Without Th2 cells, you wouldn't activate the B cells.
Activated T cytotoxic cells divide and go out into the blood. They circulate through the body, looking for cells that are making the antigen. A cell that's infected with a virus will display the viral antigen on MHC-I proteins. When T cytotoxic cells find an antigen they recognize on a cell's MHC-I proteins, they kill that cell. This is part of CELL-MEDIATED IMMUNITY.	If you didn't have T cytotoxic cells, you wouldn't be as able to fight off viral infections.
Th2 cells activate B cells that recognize the antigen. The B cells divide and some of them become plasma cells. These produce ANTIBODIES or IMMUNOGLOBULINS, which are proteins designed to attach to the antigen. This is called HUMORAL IMMUNITY.	Without B cells or antibodies, it would be hard for you to fight off infections or to prevent them. This would especially apply to bacterial infections and parasites.
Antibodies can make antigens stick together, mark them for white blood cells to eat, or cause a group of poisonous proteins in your blood called COMPLEMENT to destroy them. They can also attach to Mast cells and make the Mast cells respond to the antigen.	If you didn't have enough complement, you would have trouble killing many antigens. If your complement turned on at the wrong time or in the wrong place, it might damage your own tissues.

Even after you have cleared away the infection, some activated B and T cells will remain in your body as MEMORY CELLS, to protect you if you encounter the disease again. The level of antibodies in your blood may remain elevated, as well. The test measuring the levels is called an ANTIBODY TITER. These remaining antibodies can stop you from getting infected again with the disease.	If you didn't have memory cells and circulating antibodies, the next time you encountered that disease it would have a second chance to infect you while the immune system was responding to it. This is why you get periodic booster shots. A booster shot contains antigens that stimulate the B memory cells to make antibodies, so your antibody titer goes up and you're already protected against a disease when you encounter it.

Bigley, V., Barge, D., & Collin, M. (2016). Dendritic cell analysis in primary immunodeficiency. Current Opinion in Allergy and Clinical Immunology, 16(6), 530–540. http://www.ncbi.nlm.nih.gov/pmc/articles/PMC5087571/

Reith, W., & Mach, B. (2001). The bare lymphocyte syndrome and the regulation of MHC expression. Annual Review of Immunology, 19, 331–373. https://www.ncbi.nlm.nih.gov/pubmed/11244040

Test yourself! Immune System and Immune Disorders

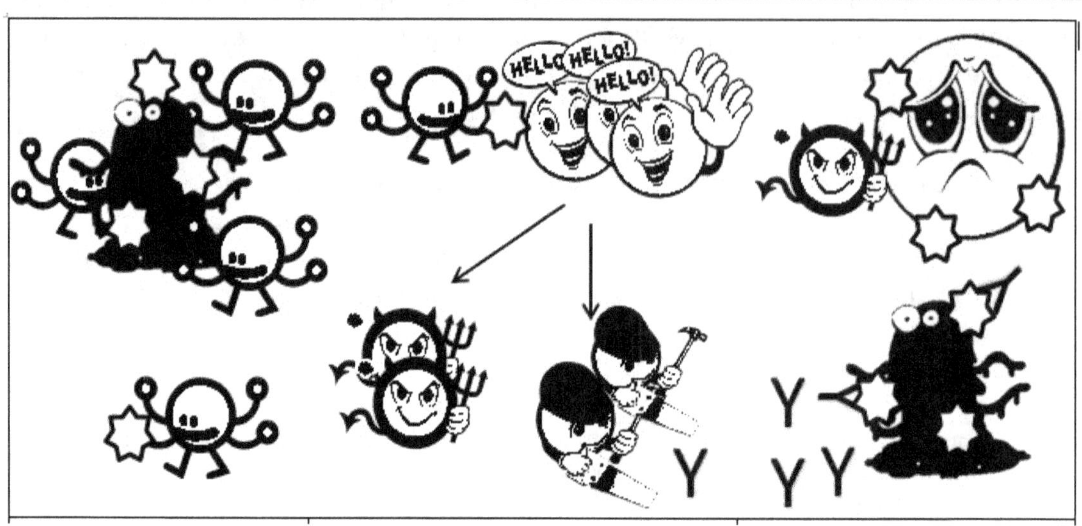

Here's a horrible virus attacking your tissues! You can identify it by the ________________ on its surface.
It begins an inflammation, which attracts ____________________ cells.
They eat the pathogen and display the ________________ on their _________proteins.

Now these _________ will enter a lymph vessel and travel up to the ____________________, where they will present the ____________________ to the immune cells, or ____________________.

Here we are in the lymph node, and the ________________ cells (also called CD4+) are looking at the ________________. If one of them has a receptor that matches it, that CD4+ cell will begin to divide and secrete ____________. It will activate the ____________________ cells and the _____ cells that have the same receptor, and start them dividing too.

The ________________ cells, also known as CD8+, will go out into the blood searching for cells making the ____________.
They will look for it on the _________ proteins on the surfaces of your cells.

The _____ cells will create special proteins that can attach to the ________________. These proteins are called ____________________ or ____________________.

Here's a poor sick cell infected with the virus. See the viral ____________ on its ____________ proteins?
When the ________________ cell detects that, it will kill this infected cell.

Meanwhile, any viruses outside the cell are being attacked by the ________________.
They will mark the virus to be eaten by ________________ or destroyed by the protein ________________.
Soon you're well! And if you meet this virus again, you have ________________ and ________________ just waiting to destroy it.

Images from Microsoft Clip Art, 2013.

Apply it! Inflammation, Immune System and Immune Disorders

Mrs. V retired to her dream home in the country, but she ran into trouble as soon as spring came and the trees bloomed. "All it took was one whiff of pollen, and my nose turned into a fountain!" she says. "Antihistamines are my new drug of choice."
What is making her nose run, and how do antihistamines relieve it?

Blood tests showed that Mrs. V had high levels of anti-birch pollen antibodies in her blood. She doesn't understand how these got there. How did she develop these antibodies, and how did they begin an inflammation?

The birch trees stopped blooming, and Mrs. V got out in the backyard. There, she discovered a new problem – poison ivy! Her backyard was full of it, and even though she wore gloves and was very careful while she cleared it out, she got a rash. She complained to her doctor about this allergy that was making her sick over and over. "This isn't the same allergy," the doctor said. "For one thing, the antigen you're reacting against is different. For another, this rash is caused by T cytotoxic cells, not by antibodies."
What are T cytotoxic cells, how did she get them, and how are they causing a rash?

The Bridge Between – Hemostasis and Clotting Disorders

Normal clotting (hemostasis)	What if it Goes Wrong?
So, you hurt yourself. The damaged cells will release inflammatory mediators, compounds that start an inflammation. These include thromboxane A2, which activates platelet aggregation, making platelets clump together.	If you didn't make thromboxane A2, you would have decreased clotting. This is one reason aspirin is often prescribed for people who are at risk of strokes, because it reduces thromboxane A2 production.
Platelets or Thrombocytes are not cells. They are fragments of cells called megakaryocytes. They are made in your bone marrow.	If your bone marrow weren't making platelets fast enough, you would have trouble clotting as quickly as usual. If you made too many platelets, you might clot too much.
Platelet production is controlled by the hormone THROMBOPOIETIN, which is made in your liver and kidneys. When THROMBOPOIETIN is released into the blood, it can travel to the bone marrow and stimulate platelet formation.	If you couldn't make adequate THROMBOPOIETIN, your platelet count would decrease and you might have too much bleeding (Wörmann, 2013).
The amount of platelet formation depends on how much THROMBOPOIETIN reaches the bone marrow. If you already have platelets in your blood, they trap the THROMBOPOIETIN and keep some of it from reaching the bone marrow.	If platelets didn't trap the THROMBOPOIETIN, all of it would reach your bone marrow and you would keep making platelets even when you had enough. You might develop excessive clotting (though I could not find a disease with this mechanism, so this is speculation).
Platelets circulate in your blood until they reach a damaged area. Then they use a protein called von Willebrand factor to attach to collagen at the injury site.	If your blood were moving more slowly, it would be easier for platelets to attach and form a clot. If you couldn't make enough von Willebrand factor, the platelets wouldn't attach as well and you would take longer to clot.
After a platelet attaches to the injured area, it releases compounds, including thromboxane A2, which attract more platelets, help them stick to one another, cause the blood vessel to constrict, and promote clotting.	If there weren't enough of these compounds, it would be harder to clot (World Federation of Hemophilia, 2012). Aspirin blocks a platelet's ability to make thromboxane A2, so it reduces clotting.

A clot requires more than platelets. It requires a network of fibrin proteins to bind the platelets together. The fibrin proteins are made out of fibrinogen proteins circulating in the blood.	If you didn't have enough fibrinogen, you wouldn't be able to clot as quickly as usual.
Fibrinogen is converted to fibrin by an enzyme called thrombin. Thrombin is made from circulating prothrombin.	If you didn't have enough prothrombin, you wouldn't be able to clot as quickly as usual.
A large number of procoagulation factors are needed to activate thrombin. Many of them are proteins made in the liver.	If you were deficient in any of these procoagulation factors, you would not be able to clot as quickly as usual.
The liver requires Vitamin K to synthesize many of the procoagulation factors.	If you didn't have enough Vitamin K, you would not be able to clot as quickly as usual.
Calcium is needed for many procoagulation factors to work.	If you didn't have enough calcium, you wouldn't be able to clot as quickly as usual (Morotti *et al.*, 2016).
Procoagulation factors are activated by two major events: when the blood comes into contact with injured blood vessels (the intrinsic system) or when the blood comes in contact with fluid from damaged tissues (the extrinsic system).	If a lot of fluid from damaged tissues got into the blood, or there was widespread damage to the blood vessel lining, you might start forming lots of clots.
Anticoagulation factors help regulate clot formation and keep it from happening too much. The liver produces many of these compounds.	If your anticoagulation factors were too active, you wouldn't be able to clot as quickly as usual. If they weren't active enough, you would create too many clots.
The enzyme plasmin breaks down fibrin strands and removes the clot. Plasmin is made from the protein plasminogen.	If you didn't have enough plasminogen, you would not be able to break down clots effectively.
Tissue plasminogen activator turns the plasminogen into plasmin, which then breaks down the clot.	If you had more tissue plasminogen activator, your clots would break down faster. That's why it is used as a clot-busting treatment for people with strokes.

Morotti, A., Charidimou, A., Phuah, C.-L., Jessel, M. J., Schwab, K., Ayres, A. M., … Goldstein, J. N. (2016). Association Between Serum Calcium Level and Extent of Bleeding in Patients With Intracerebral Hemorrhage. JAMA Neurology, 73(11), 1285–1290. https://doi.org/10.1001/jamaneurol.2016.2252

World Federation of Hemophilia. (2012, May). Storage pool deficiencies. Retrieved March 17, 2017, from https://www.wfh.org/en/page.aspx?pid=655

Wörmann, B. (2013). Clinical Indications for Thrombopoietin and Thrombopoietin-Receptor Agonists. *Transfusion Medicine and Hemotherapy*, 40(5), 319–325. https://doi.org/10.1159/000355006

Test yourself! Hemostasis and Clotting Disorders

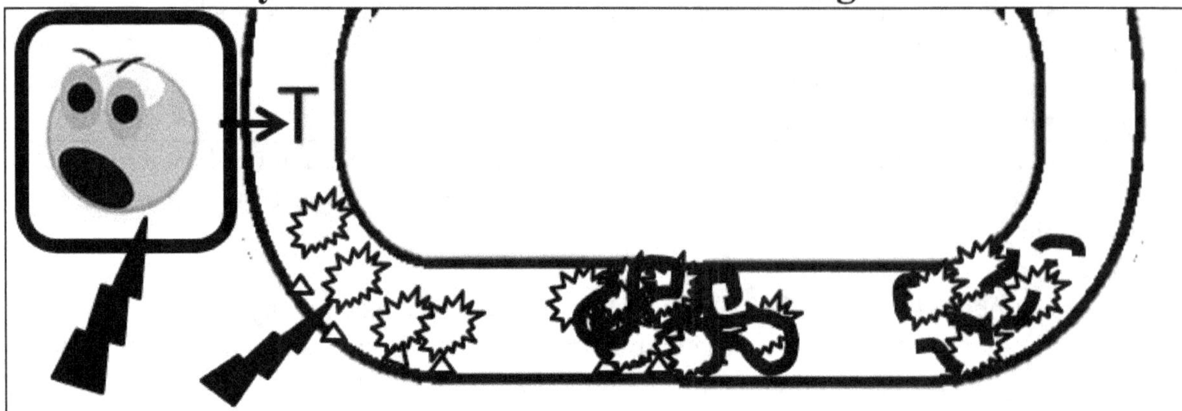

Here's your poor sad cell, damaged by some awful trauma!
The cell will create inflammatory mediators. These include __________________, which increases platelet function.

Your blood vessel has been damaged too. Some of its cells are broken, and the collagen underneath is showing through.

Platelets, or __________________, attach to the damaged area. They need __________________ factor to attach to collagen.

Compounds from the injured blood vessel (the __________________ system) and from damaged tissues (the ______________ system) activate __________________ factors in the bloodstream. Many of these are proteins that were synthesized by the ________________. Vitamin _______ is needed to synthesize them, and ____________ is needed for them to work.

The __________________ factors activate the enzyme ___________________, which turns __________________ in the blood into ___________ filaments. These filaments then tie the platelets together into a strong clot.

Clot production is kept from going too far by __________________ factors made in the liver.

The clot breaks down when tissue __________________ activator turns the blood protein __________________ into the enzyme ________________, which breaks the ___________ strands apart.

Sad cell from Microsoft clip art, 2013

Apply it! Hemostasis and Clotting Disorders

Mr. G is in the hospital because of complications associated with liver and kidney failure. His blood results are way off; he has high levels of waste products in his blood, very low platelet and erythrocyte counts, and low calcium.

The doctors are discussing whether he should be put on dialysis to clean the wastes out of his blood.

Doctor Bob says, "I'm worried about his bleeding too much." Why is Dr. Bob worried about bleeding?

Doctor Sue says, "There's recent work suggesting that liver failure can cause too much clotting, though." How could liver failure increase clotting?

"That's true," says Dr. Bob, "but his med history shows that he's also been taking a lot of aspirin." Why is this relevant?

The Bridge Between – Red Blood Cells and Anemias

Normal Red Blood Cell Physiology	What if it Goes Wrong?
To keep a normal amount of red blood cells (erythrocytes) in your circulation, you need to keep a balance between how many you make and how many you destroy. Erythrocytes are made in your red bone marrow.	If something went wrong with your bone marrow, you might not be able to make enough erythrocytes. This is called aplastic anemia.
If there isn't enough oxygen reaching your tissues, the kidneys respond by secreting the hormone ERYTHROPOIETIN. This travels to the bone marrow and tells it to make more erythrocytes.	If your kidneys weren't working, you wouldn't be able to make enough ERYTHROPOIETIN and your bone marrow wouldn't create enough erythrocytes.
The immature RBCs in the bone marrow have organelles like other cells, but as they mature they lose those organelles and fill up with hemoglobin, the oxygen-carrying pigment. The immature RBCs lose their nuclei and most organelles and become reticulocytes. Then the reticulocytes are released into the blood. They lose their endoplasmic reticulum and become mature RBCs or erythrocytes.	Hemoglobin requires iron, so if you didn't have enough iron your RBCs would not be full of hemoglobin and wouldn't be able to carry enough oxygen. RBC maturation in the bone marrow requires folic acid and Vitamin B12. Without enough of these nutrients, you would be less able to make mature RBCs. If the bone marrow had to replace RBCs too fast, the blood would contain more immature RBCs – reticulocytes or even some that still had their nuclei!
RBCs circulate in the blood for about 120 days, or until they become too damaged for the spleen to repair.	If something damaged the RBCs, they wouldn't circulate for as long as usual before being destroyed. They might be destroyed faster than they could be replaced, causing anemia.
Old or damaged RBCs are trapped in the spleen, where the heme portion of the hemoglobin inside them can be processed into a less toxic compound, bilirubin.	If the RBCs were to break outside the spleen, the hemoglobin would spill out into the plasma. If the spleen were too big and active (hypersplenism), it might break down more RBCs than necessary (Brill & Baumgardner, 2000). If the spleen broke down too many RBCs, you might get too much bilirubin in the blood and develop jaundice.
The bilirubin circulates in your blood until it reaches the liver. The liver removes it and uses it to help make bile, which is stored in the gall bladder.	If the liver weren't working fast enough, the excess bilirubin might deposit in your skin, eyes, and other tissues.

John R. Brill, & Baumgardner, D. J. (2000). Normocytic Anemia. American Family Physician, 62(10), 2255–2263.

Test yourself! Red Blood Cells and Anemias

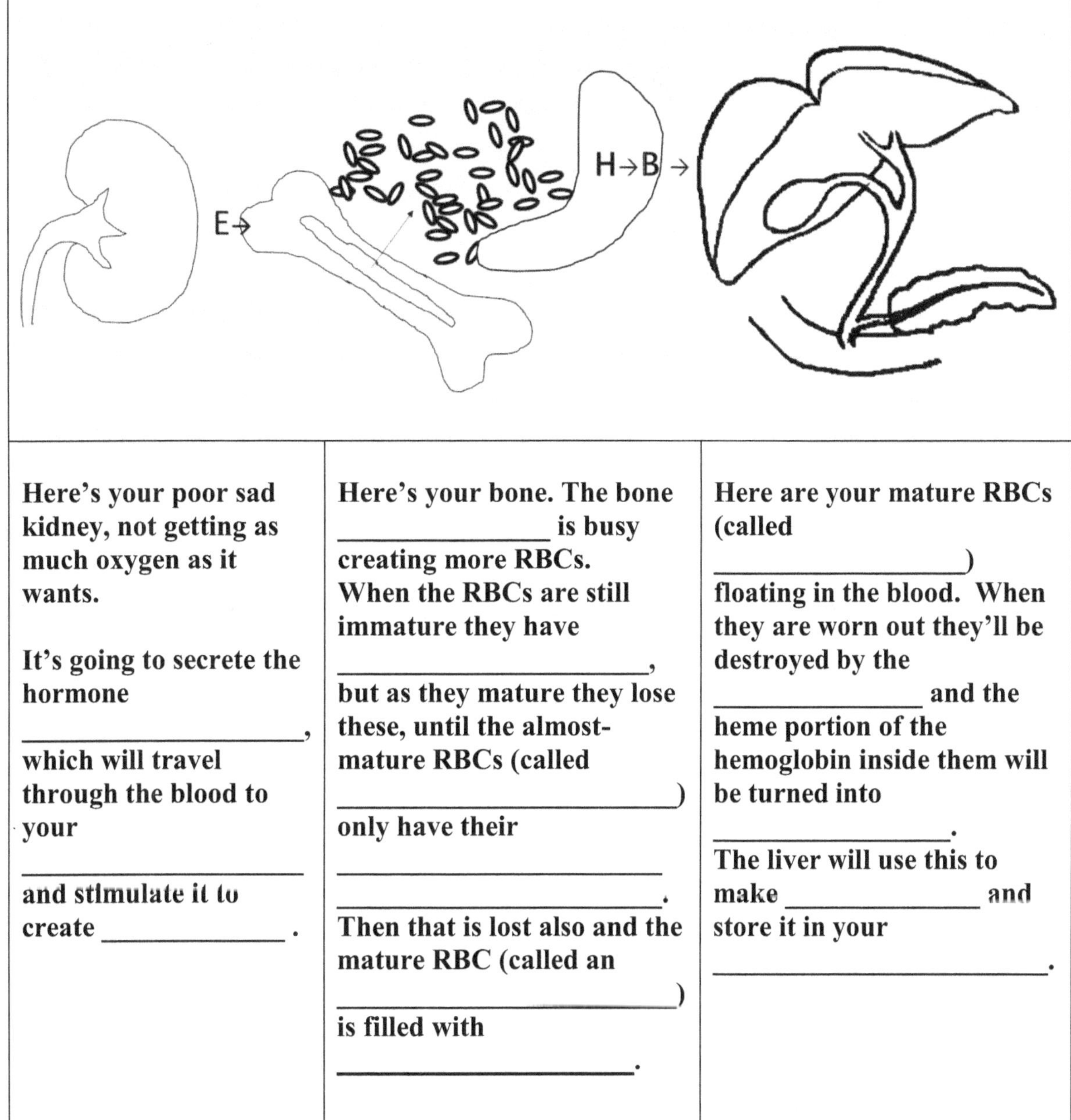

Here's your poor sad kidney, not getting as much oxygen as it wants.

It's going to secrete the hormone

__________________,

which will travel through the blood to your

____

and stimulate it to create __________ .

Here's your bone. The bone __________________ is busy creating more RBCs. When the RBCs are still immature they have

__________________,

but as they mature they lose these, until the almost-mature RBCs (called

__________________)

only have their

____

__________________.

Then that is lost also and the mature RBC (called an

__________________)

is filled with

__________________.

Here are your mature RBCs (called

__________________)

floating in the blood. When they are worn out they'll be destroyed by the

__________________ and the heme portion of the hemoglobin inside them will be turned into

__________________.

The liver will use this to make __________ and store it in your

__________________.

Apply it! Red Blood Cells and Anemias

Mr. A has an inherited condition that damages the membranes on his RBCs, causing them to develop an abnormal shape and wear out too quickly. Why has he developed anemia?

The doctor is checking Mr. A's liver and spleen. Why does the doctor expect them to be enlarged?

Now the doctor has ordered blood tests for erythrocytes, reticulocytes, and ERYTHROPOIETIN. What do you expect the results to be like? Why?

The Bridge Between – Osmosis and Fluid Imbalance

Normal Water balance	What if it Goes Wrong?
You take in water by drinking it. Normally you become thirsty when cells in your hypothalamus dehydrate and begin to shrink. When you rehydrate yourself, these cells pick up water and return to their normal size. Then you aren't thirsty any more.	If you couldn't drink you would become dehydrated. If people didn't respond to the shrinking hypothalamus cells, they might not drink enough water and become chronically dehydrated. This blunted thirst response is more common in older people. People who didn't stop drinking when their cells were back to normal could develop brain swelling.
Water moves through the semipermeable membranes of your cells by osmosis. That is, it moves from areas where there is mostly water (HYPOTONIC) to areas where there is less water and more solutes (HYPERTONIC). The easy way to remember this: WATER FOLLOWS SOLUTES.	If your blood became very dilute, or hypotonic, then water would move from the blood into your cells and make them swell. If your blood became very concentrated, or hypertonic, then water would move from your cells into your blood and cells would shrink.
After you drink water, you must absorb it from your GI contents into your blood. There is no 'pump' to move water; your body has to move solutes, and the water follows them by osmosis. Remember: WATER FOLLOWS SOLUTES! The small intestine absorbs food from your GI tract into your blood, and the water in your GI tract follows the solutes into your blood.	If you couldn't absorb solutes from the gut contents into the blood, the water would also stay in the gut contents. In fact, if the gut contents had a higher concentration of solutes than the blood, water would move from the blood into the gut contents. If the small intestine couldn't digest the food, or if it couldn't absorb the food into the blood, the food and water would remain in the intestine and be lost in the stools.
The large intestine absorbs ions from the GI contents into the blood. Water follows the ions by osmosis.	If the large intestine didn't absorb ions, or if it secreted them instead, water wouldn't be absorbed into the blood either and the ions and water would be lost in the stools.
Once you have absorbed water into your blood, it circulates in your blood vessels. Blood pressure pushes some of it out of the small vessels into your tissues, sort of like a soaker hose[1]. This fluid ends up in the INTERCELLULAR SPACE (between the cells) in your tissues.	If too much water were pushed out of the vessels into the tissues, your tissues would start to swell up with fluid -- edema. This is one reason people who have high blood pressure could develop swollen feet. Because it was blood pressure that pushed the water out into the tissue, you could counteract it by applying an opposing pressure with pressure stockings.

As the blood vessels passing through your tissues lose water, the blood inside them becomes more hypertonic, so at the end of the tissue some water moves back into them by osmosis. Not all of it, though! The remaining fluid is removed from the tissues by lymph vessels, which carry it up to lymph nodes. It is then returned to the blood.	If lymph vessels were blocked or lymph nodes removed, the fluid would have a harder time getting out of the tissue and you might develop swelling -- lymphedema.
Water is always moving between the blood, the intercellular space, and your cells by the combined forces of blood pressure, lymphatic flow, and osmosis.	The more permeable your capillaries are, the faster water can move into tissues. This is how inflammation causes local swelling.
You can lose water by evaporation from your skin – sweat. It also evaporates from your lungs every time you exhale.	Someone who was hot or breathing heavily would lose more water this way.
The main way you balance water, though, is to send it out in your urine.	If your kidneys didn't work, you wouldn't be able to regulate your water balance.
If your body is dehydrated, the cells in your hypothalamus will secrete ANTIDIURETIC HORMONE (ADH, also called VASOPRESSIN). This hormone makes the nephrons in your kidneys more permeable to water, so water in the urine can move into your blood by osmosis and correct the dehydration.	If you couldn't make ADH, you wouldn't be able to reabsorb water from your urine sufficiently. You'd always be urinating, and would have to keep drinking to avoid dehydration. If you made too much ADH, you'd always be moving water from your urine into your blood, and your blood might become too dilute (HYPOTONIC). Then your cells would swell.
If blood pressure decreases, your kidneys will begin the renin-angiotensin-ALDOSTERONE system (RAAS). ALDOSTERONE makes your kidneys run the Na^+/K^+ ATPase, a pump which moves 3 Na^+ from the urine into the blood and 2K^+ from the blood into the urine. Because water follows the majority of solutes, it will move from the urine to the blood. WATCH OUT – this system is putting Na^+ AND water into your blood. So while it's increasing your blood VOLUME, it isn't really changing your blood osmolarity. This isn't a way to water down your blood.	If you couldn't run the RAAS, you'd have trouble reabsorbing water and Na^+ and maintaining your blood volume. You'd also have trouble getting K^+ out of your blood. If you ran the RAAS too much, you'd move too much Na^+ and water into your blood and develop high blood pressure. And you'd be losing your K^+ in the urine.

1.a garden hose with tiny holes in it, so water can seep out onto the ground and water the plants slowly.

Test yourself! Osmosis and Fluid Imbalance

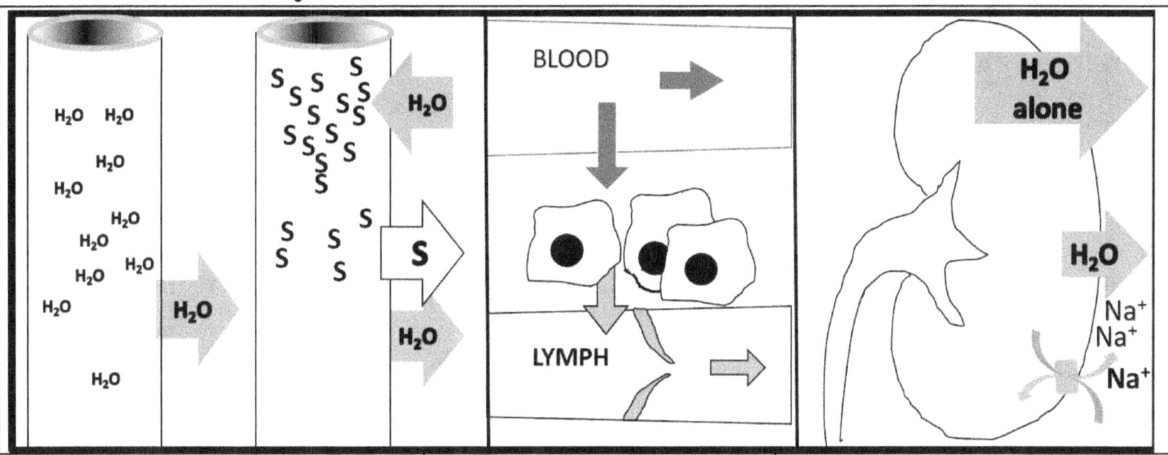

Here's the water you drank, in your GI tract. It can only get into your blood by ______________.
That's easy if all you did was drink, because drinking water made your GI contents ________tonic to your blood, and water will move _________ the blood.

If you ate food as well, your GI contents contains solutes (S) and may be _________tonic to your blood. Then water will move from the __________ into the ______________.
As your small intestine absorbs the food into the blood, water will ____________ the food solutes back into the blood.

In the large intestine, you'll absorb _________ from the GI contents into the blood. Water will _________ those solutes too, ending up in the _________.

Here's a blood vessel flowing through your tissue. As your blood passes through tissues, ________________ pushes some of the water out of the vessel into the ______________ space.

If too much water enters the ______________ space, that tissue could develop ________________.
But water is removed by the _________ vessel at the bottom of the picture, which sends it to the __________________ and then back into the venous blood.
Finally, water from your blood filters into the urine in your kidneys.

If your body is dehydrated, cells in your hypothalamus will _________. This stimulates the hypothalamus to start the ____________ response and to secrete __________, a hormone which makes your kidneys reabsorb water into your blood.
The water added to your blood will make the blood ______________ and the hypothalamus cells will ___________, shutting off the response.
Water can also be reabsorbed from the kidneys by the ______ system, which activates ________ ATPase. This protein moves ___________from the blood into the urine and ___________ from the urine into the blood. Water follows the _______ back into the blood, increasing blood _____________.

Apply it! Osmosis and fluid balance

Mr. D has diabetes insipidus – he can't make ADH. How will this affect his ability to control blood osmolarity?

One of the side effects of diabetes insipidus is constant thirst. How is the disorder leading to this effect?

Another side effect of diabetes insipidus is constant urination. Mr. D has this too! How was it caused?

Mr. D has been coping with his disease very well, just by adjusting his behavior. But then he caught the 'stomach flu' and spent two days sick in bed. He says he was barely able to get to the toilet fast enough to throw up. He ran a high fever and his respiration rate increased, as well. Then he had cold sweats. Right now he says he feels horrible, and when you check his vitals you see that his eyes are sunken, his lips are dry, his pulse is rapid and weak and his blood pressure is dangerously low. What has happened to his water balance, and why?

Mr. D's wife had the same 'stomach flu,' but although she threw up just as much and had the same fever, her blood pressure is almost normal. Why?

The Bridge Between – Potassium and Potassium Imbalance

Normal Potassium (K^+) Physiology	What if it Goes Wrong?
You get K^+ by eating it.	If you didn't eat enough, you wouldn't get enough. You'd develop a K^+ deficit.
After you eat it, you must absorb it from your intestines into your blood.	If you couldn't absorb K^+ from your diet, it would go out in the stools and you would develop a K^+ deficit (Penn State Hershey Medical Center, 2015).
Once you have absorbed the K^+ into your blood, most of it moves into your cells.	If cells were broken by crushing injuries, chemotherapy, or other damage, they would release the K^+ into the blood. This would cause K^+ excess, or hyperkalemia.
K^+ is moved into your cells by ion pumps, including the Na^+/K^+ ATPase protein in your cell membranes. This protein uses ATP for energy. For every ATP, it moves 2 K^+ into the cell and 3 Na^+ out of the cell. The Na^+/K^+ ATPase is activated by INSULIN and the Sympathetic Nervous System (SNS, mainly via Beta receptors).	If you couldn't make INSULIN, you would have trouble moving K^+ from your blood into your cells. You might develop high blood K^+ (Liamis *et al.*, 2014). If you took too much INSULIN, or took beta-agonist drugs to increase SNS function, you might move too much K^+ into your cells and develop low blood K^+ (Castro and Sharma, 2019).
Cells can also pick up K^+ from the blood in exchange for H^+. They can run this exchange either way: they can use it to pick up K^+ and release H^+ into the blood, or to pick up H^+ and release K^+ into the blood.	If your cells used this exchange to correct the blood levels of K^+, they would change the blood levels of H^+ and the blood pH. If they used this exchange to correct blood levels of H^+, that would change the blood K^+ levels.
K+ can diffuse out of the cell through K+ channels, due to the concentration gradient between the blood and the cell.	When blood K+ rises, less K+ will diffuse out of the cell. When blood K+ decreases, more K+ will diffuse out of the cell.
K^+ filters from the blood into your urine	As long as your kidneys were working right, you would probably not get high blood K^+. But if your kidneys failed, it would be a likely problem.
Much of the K^+ is reabsorbed from the urine into your blood.	If you produce urine too fast for the K^+ to be reabsorbed, you might lose a lot of K^+.
If your blood K^+ is too high, your adrenal cortex will secrete ALDOSTERONE, activating the Na^+/K^+ ATPase in your kidneys to pump $3Na^+$ from urine to blood and $2K^+$ from blood into urine. This will lower your blood K^+.	A person with too much ALDOSTERONE would lose too much K^+ in their urine. A person without enough ALDOSTERONE would keep too much K^+ in their blood.

The level of K$^+$ in your blood controls your cells' electric charge, or RESTING POTENTIAL. Normal resting potential is around -90 mV.	If blood K$^+$ increased, resting potential would become more positive – for example, it might move up from -90 mV to -70 mV. This cell would be hypopolarized. If blood K$^+$ were lower than normal, resting potential would be lower, like –100 mV. This cell would be hyperpolarized.
For a neuron or muscle cell to fire, enough Na$^+$ must enter the cell to raise its potential to a threshold level of around -55 mV. At this charge, lots of voltage-gated Na$^+$ channel proteins change their shape to let more Na$^+$ flow into the cell, and the cell fires.	If blood K$^+$ were too high, resting potential would increase and be nearer threshold. The cell would become extra sensitive and react to tiny stimuli. It might eventually fire and not be able to re-set itself – then it would stop working entirely. If blood K$^+$ were too low, the resting potential would move down, farther away from threshold. This cell might not respond very well, because it would take a very large stimulus to let in enough Na$^+$ to get its charge up to threshold.

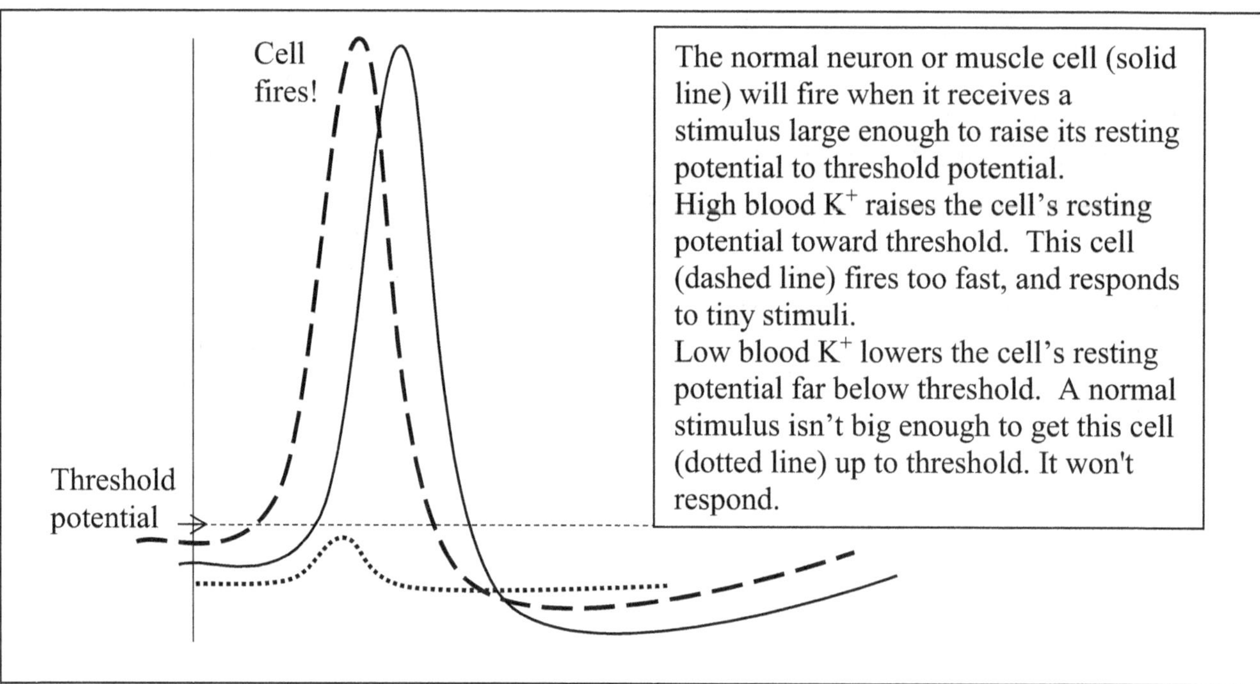

The normal neuron or muscle cell (solid line) will fire when it receives a stimulus large enough to raise its resting potential to threshold potential.

High blood K$^+$ raises the cell's resting potential toward threshold. This cell (dashed line) fires too fast, and responds to tiny stimuli.

Low blood K$^+$ lowers the cell's resting potential far below threshold. A normal stimulus isn't big enough to get this cell (dotted line) up to threshold. It won't respond.

Castro, D., & Sharma, S. (2019). Hypokalemia. In *StatPearls*. Retrieved from http://www.ncbi.nlm.nih.gov/books/NBK482465/

Liamis, G., Liberopoulos, E., Barkas, F., & Elisaf, M. (2014). Diabetes mellitus and electrolyte disorders. World Journal of Clinical Cases : WJCC, 2(10), 488–496. https://doi.org/10.12998/wjcc.v2.i10.488

Penn State Hershey Medical Center. (2015, August 5). Potassium. Retrieved March 21, 2017, from http://pennstatehershey.adam.com/content.aspx?productId=107&pid=33&gid=000320

Test yourself! Potassium and Potassium Imbalance

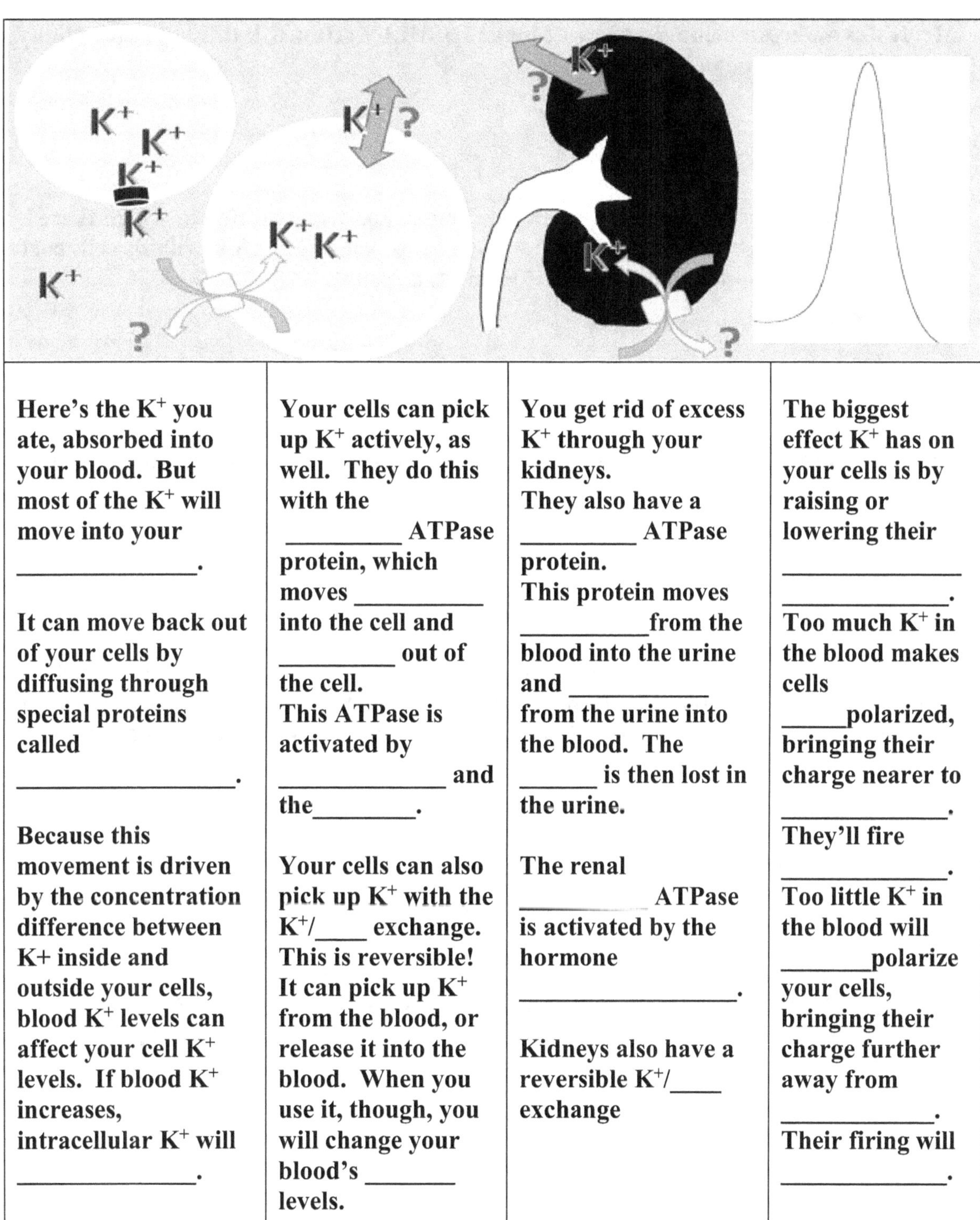

Here's the K+ you ate, absorbed into your blood. But most of the K+ will move into your _____________.

It can move back out of your cells by diffusing through special proteins called ________________.

Because this movement is driven by the concentration difference between K+ inside and outside your cells, blood K+ levels can affect your cell K+ levels. If blood K+ increases, intracellular K+ will _____________.

Your cells can pick up K+ actively, as well. They do this with the __________ ATPase protein, which moves __________ into the cell and __________ out of the cell.
This ATPase is activated by _____________ and the________.

Your cells can also pick up K+ with the K+/____ exchange. This is reversible! It can pick up K+ from the blood, or release it into the blood. When you use it, though, you will change your blood's _______ levels.

You get rid of excess K+ through your kidneys.
They also have a __________ ATPase protein.
This protein moves __________ from the blood into the urine and __________ from the urine into the blood. The _______ is then lost in the urine.

The renal __________ ATPase is activated by the hormone ________________.

Kidneys also have a reversible K+/____ exchange

The biggest effect K+ has on your cells is by raising or lowering their _____________.

Too much K+ in the blood makes cells _____polarized, bringing their charge nearer to _____________.

They'll fire _____________.

Too little K+ in the blood will _______polarize your cells, bringing their charge further away from _____________.

Their firing will _____________.

Apply it! Potassium and Potassium Imbalance

Mr. K has diabetes mellitus – he can't make INSULIN. How will this affect his ability to move K^+ from his blood into his cells?

One of the side effects of diabetes mellitus is ketoacidosis, a condition in which there is too much H^+ in the blood. Mr. K has developed this condition. How will his cells correct it, and what will happen to his blood K^+ levels as a result?

Another side effect of diabetes mellitus is kidney failure. Mr. K has this too! How will it affect his blood K^+ levels?

Mr. K is feeling very strange. Sometimes his heart feels like it's missing beats, and sometimes his legs cramp up. The doctor ordered an EKG and when it came back, she was really concerned. She said his heart wasn't firing normally. How could his K^+ levels be involved in this?

The doctor treated Mr. K with INSULIN. The med student wanted to know if they shouldn't give him some ALDOSTERONE to fix his K^+ levels, but the doctor said INSULIN would be enough. Would ALDOSTERONE have been a good idea?

The Bridge Between – Calcium and Calcium Imbalance

Normal calcium Physiology	What if it Goes Wrong?
You get calcium by eating it.	If you didn't eat enough calcium, you would have to use the calcium stored in your bones.
After you eat it, you must absorb it from your intestines into your blood.	If you couldn't absorb it, calcium would go out in your stools and you would have to use the calcium stored in your bones.
To absorb calcium from your diet, you need activated VITAMIN D3.	Without activated VITAMIN D3, you would not be able to absorb calcium and it would just go out in your stools.
You can get VITAMIN D3 from your diet, but it is a fat-soluble vitamin.	If you couldn't digest fats, you would have trouble absorbing enough VITAMIN D3.
You can make VITAMIN D3 in your skin, if you're exposed to UV light or sunlight	If you weren't exposed to enough UV light or sunlight, you wouldn't make enough VITAMIN D3.
Whether it comes from your diet or from your skin, the VITAMIN D3 must be activated in your liver and then your kidneys before it will work.	If your kidneys had stopped working, you wouldn't activate enough VITAMIN D3. You would have trouble absorbing calcium.
Once you have absorbed the calcium into your blood, about half of it binds to proteins and other molecules in the blood. This calcium doesn't directly affect your cells. The other half of the calcium circulates as ionized calcium, or Ca^{2+}. This ion can have different effects on different cells.	Be careful when you read the patient's chart! Did they measure total calcium or ionized calcium?
If Ca^{2+} is outside the cells, in the blood, it can block Na^+ channels on nerve and skeletal muscle cells (Armstrong & Cota, 1991). Blocking these channels reduces the cells' ability to fire.	If there were too much Ca^{2+} in the blood, it would block too many Na^+ channels and decrease nerve and skeletal muscle firing, causing weakness If there were too little Ca^{2+} in the blood, the nerves and skeletal muscles would be able to fire too much, causing cramps and spasms
Some cells (like cardiac muscle and smooth muscle) have Ca^{2+} channels that allow Ca^{2+} to enter the cells. Once it's inside, it helps with cell contraction (Catterall, 2015; Godfraind, 2014).	The more Ca^{2+} you have in the blood, the more smooth and cardiac cells can contract. People who need to decrease their cardiac and smooth muscle contraction (to lower blood pressure, for instance) might take calcium channel blockers to keep the calcium from getting into their cells.

Calcium in the blood is also necessary for clotting factors to work.	If you didn't have enough calcium in the blood, you wouldn't clot fast enough. You might develop bruising and bleeding.
Calcium in the blood can be moved into the bones.	If you had a calcium deficit, you move less calcium into your bones and they would gradually become weaker.
The hormones THYROCALCITONIN (or CALCITONIN) and ESTROGEN help stimulate bone cells to pick up calcium from the blood	People with less ESTROGEN (postmenopausal women) release more calcium from their bones, move less into their bones, and are at greater risk of osteoporosis.
Weight-bearing exercise also causes the bone cells to pick up calcium from the blood	Patients who are bedridden or mobility impaired have a harder time moving calcium into their bones.
Calcium in the blood can also be filtered into the urine	People who had high blood calcium could develop kidney stones from the large amount of calcium moved into their urine.
If you don't have enough calcium in your blood, your parathyroid glands will release PARATHYROID HORMONE (PTH) to raise blood calcium levels.	If your parathyroids had been removed or didn't work, you would have trouble keeping blood calcium levels high enough.
PARATHYROID HORMONE helps you absorb calcium from your diet by increasing the amount of Vit D activated by your kidneys.	Without PARATHYROID HORMONE, you'd activate less Vit D and be less able to absorb calcium from your diet or reabsorb it from your urine.
When PARATHYROID HORMONE is first released, it stimulates the bone-building cells. But that changes if the PARATHYROID HORMONE levels stay high.	Giving someone a single injection of PARATHYROID HORMONE every day would strengthen their bones! It's a treatment for osteoporosis (Rubin & Bilezikian, 2002).
If PARATHYROID HORMONE levels STAY high, they cause your bone cells to release calcium from the bones into the blood.	Without PARATHYROID HORMONE, the bones wouldn't release calcium into the blood and blood calcium levels might remain too low. With too much PARATHYROID HORMONE, the bones would release too much calcium into the blood and the blood calcium might become too high. The bones might become weak and easy to break.

Armstrong, C. M., & Cota, G. (1991). Calcium ion as a cofactor in Na channel gating. Proceedings of the National Academy of Sciences of the United States of America, 88(15), 6528–6531.
Catterall, W. A. (2015). Regulation of Cardiac Calcium Channels in the Fight-or-Flight Response. Current Molecular Pharmacology, 8(1), 12–21. https://www.ncbi.nlm.nih.gov/pmc/articles/PMC4664455/
Godfraind, T. (2014). Calcium channel blockers in cardiovascular pharmacotherapy. Journal of Cardiovascular Pharmacology and Therapeutics, 19(6), 501–515. https://doi.org/10.1177/1074248414530508
Rubin, M. R., & Bilezikian, J. P. (2002). The potential of parathyroid hormone as a therapy for osteoporosis. International Journal of Fertility and Women's Medicine, 47(3), 103–115.

Test yourself! Calcium and Calcium Imbalance

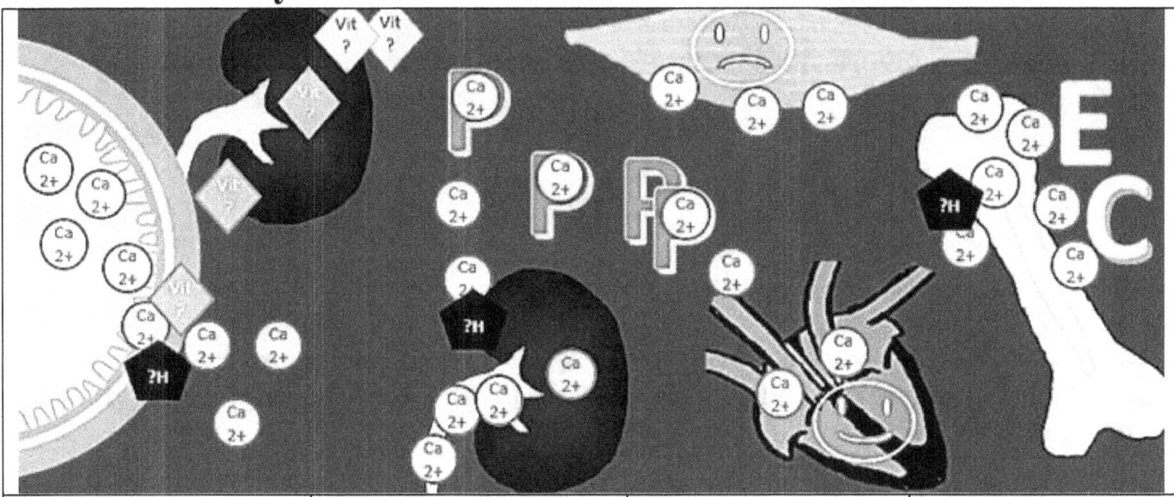

Here's your intestine, full of the dairy products you ate. If you have enough ____________ hormone and activated Vitamin _____, you can absorb the calcium from this food into your blood. You can get that Vitamin ___ from your diet if you are able to digest __________. Or you can make it in your _________, if there's enough _______________. Either way, the Vitamin ___ must be activated by your ______________ before it will help you absorb calcium from your diet.	Here are the calcium ions absorbed into your blood. About half of them will bind to ________________ The other half become the _________ ion, and are called _____________ calcium. Some of the calcium filters out of the blood into your kidneys, and is lost in your ___________. When the calcium ions attach to the outside of skeletal muscle cells, they block the ________ channels and make it harder for the muscle to fire.	But the heart and ___________ muscles have special proteins called _______________ _____________, which let the calcium into the cell. Once inside these cells, calcium will make them contract _____________. The hormones ____________ and _____________ help your bones store calcium. Load-bearing _______ does it too!	When blood calcium is low, your _____________ secrete _______. At first, this hormone stimulates the bone-building cells. If it remains elevated, though, it has a different effect. If _________ remains elevated, it will help you absorb Ca^{2+} from your intestines, reabsorb it from your urine, and release it from your bones into the blood.

Apply it! Calcium and Calcium Imbalance

Mr. P has kidney failure. How will this affect his ability to absorb calcium from his diet?

The medical student expected Mr. P to develop low blood calcium, so she did a neurological test to check. If he has low blood calcium, will he develop stronger or weaker reflexes? Why?

The medical student was surprised to find Mr. P's reflexes normal. She ordered an analysis of his blood and found that his blood calcium levels were normal! Where could he be getting the calcium to keep his blood levels normal?

The medical student ordered measurements of Mr. P's PARATHYROID HORMONE levels. Do you think they are high or low? Why?

Before the test results came back, Mr. P stubbed his toe while going to the bathroom. His foot is really sore and his toe is swollen. The medical student says this injury isn't related to his calcium balance, since his reflexes were normal. The nurse thinks it might be related. How might it be related?

The Bridge Between – Acid, Base, and Acid-Base Imbalances

Normal acid-base balance	What if it Goes Wrong?
Your body is always producing acids, as a byproduct of cellular metabolism.	If you could not remove acids as fast as you make them, your blood pH would decrease.
There are two categories of acids produced in your body. VOLATILE acid is acid that can evaporate. This is CO_2 made by aerobic respiration. CO_2 can become CARBONIC ACID by interacting with H_2O in your blood – but when it reaches your lungs, you can exhale it.	If you had trouble exhaling, CARBONIC ACID would build up in your bloodstream and your blood pH would decrease. If you exhaled too much, CARBONIC ACID levels in your blood would decrease and your blood pH would rise.
NON-VOLATILE acids are acids that can't evaporate, so they cannot be removed by your lungs. Some examples of these are sulfuric acid, hydrochloric acid, ketoacids, and lactic acid. Because they don't evaporate, these acids must be removed from your blood in other ways – mainly through the kidneys.	If you made too many nonvolatile acids (for instance, by exercising till you built up lactic acid), your blood pH would decrease.
It's important to keep blood pH stable because the H^+ ions released by acids interfere with nerve and muscle firing.	If you had too many H^+ ions (low blood pH), your nerves and muscles might fire too little. If you had very little H^+ in your blood (high blood pH), nerves and muscles might fire too easily.
Although the levels of blood acids can go up and down quickly, the pH levels don't change as fast because the H^+ from acids can attach to compounds in the blood called BUFFERS. The major BUFFER molecules in your blood are BICARBONATE IONS and proteins.	If you didn't have enough buffers, blood pH would change very rapidly and you might quickly develop acid-base imbalances. If you had a lot of acid in your blood, it might bind to a lot of the BICARBONATE molecules and you would see their level decreased on lab tests.
Your cells can also regulate the H^+ levels in your blood by picking up or releasing H^+. When cells move H^+, though, they have to exchange it for a K^+ ion. Cells use this ability to keep blood K^+ stable, as well as to regulate blood pH.	If your cells pick up H^+ from your blood, they will release K^+ into your blood. If they release H^+ into your blood, they will have to pick up K^+ from the blood in exchange. If blood K^+ were high, cells would pick it up and release H^+ into the blood. Blood pH would decrease.

You use your lungs to remove acid from the blood as well. When blood CO_2 levels increase and blood pH goes down, that stimulates you to breathe more and exhale the excess CO_2. That will bring pH back up to normal. If pH were too high or CO_2 were too low, you would breathe less until they had returned to normal levels.	If you weren't able to adjust your breathing like this, you would have trouble keeping blood pH stable.
Acids and BICARBONATE in the blood are filtered into your kidneys. Your kidneys can adjust the amount that is actually lost in the urine by reabsorbing or secreting these compounds. Kidneys generally reabsorb BICARBONATE into the blood and secrete H^+ into the urine.	The more acid there is in your blood, the more there will be in your urine. If your kidneys weren't working, acid would build up in your blood and pH would decrease.
The kidneys can also exchange H^+ for K^+. Like your cells, they use this ability to keep both H^+ and K^+ levels in the blood stable.	If blood H^+ were too high (low pH), your kidneys would move H^+ into the urine and K^+ into the blood. If your blood K^+ were too high, the kidneys would move K^+ into the urine and H^+ into the blood.

Test yourself! Acid, Base, and Acid-Base Imbalances

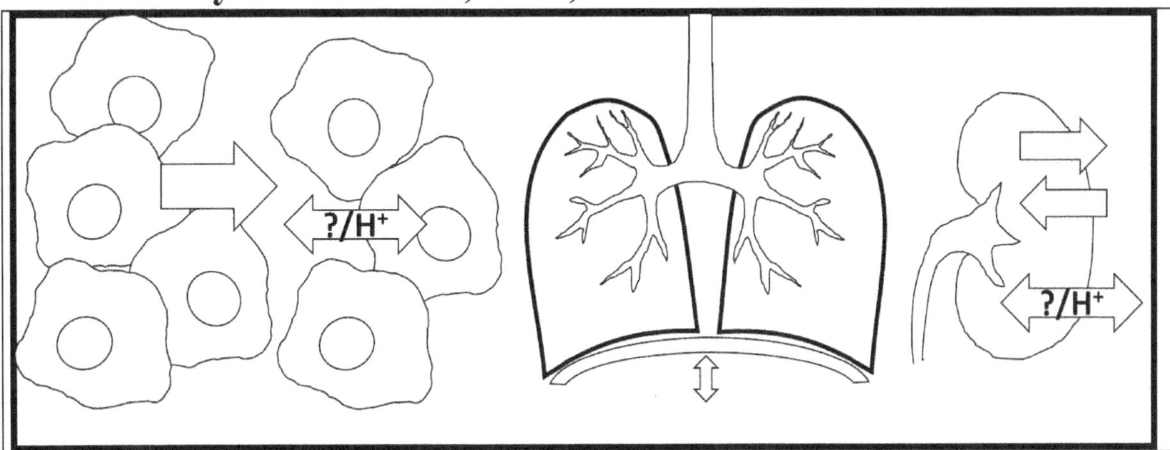

Here are your busy cells, producing all kinds of acids!

They're producing a lot of CO_2, the ______________ acid. They're also producing ____________________ acids like lactic acid, ketoacids, and hydrochloric acid.

CO_2 actually becomes an acid when it combines with __________ in the bloodstream to become ____________________________.

All these acids can affect your blood pH because they release _______ ions.

They didn't make your blood pH change too much, though, because most of those __________ ions combined with ______________ molecules in your blood. The major molecules performing this function are proteins and ____________________.

Here are your cells again, trying to regulate the acid levels in the blood.

They can do this by picking up or releasing ______ ions – but they must exchange them for _______ ions.

If your cells pick up ______ from your blood, they will release _________ into your blood.
When the blood reaches your lungs, the ____________________ breaks apart again into CO_2 and H2O. These are removed from the blood when you ____________________.
To make sure you do this enough, you regulate your breathing based on blood CO_2 and pH. You will breathe more if CO_2 is __________ or pH is _______.

Here's your kidney, filtering the acids and ______________ out of your blood.

The kidneys can raise your blood pH by sending the ___________ ions into the urine, but putting the ____________________ back into the blood.

Kidneys can also adjust blood H$^+$ by exchanging it for _______, just like your cells.

With so many ways to adjust blood pH, you manage to keep it stable. That's important because H$^+$ ions will ________________ nerve and muscle firing, if they build up in your blood.

Apply it! Acid, Base, and Acid-Base Imbalances

Mrs. T had a panic attack, which made her breathe way too fast. What happened to her blood pH? Which acid was affected, and how?

Mrs. T began to suffer some side effects from her altered blood pH. How did the panic attack change the concentration of H^+ in her blood, and what did that do to her nerves and muscles?

When her blood pH began to change, Mrs. T's cells responded to adjust it. How did that change her blood K^+ levels?

Mrs. T's kidneys also adjusted her blood pH. What were three ways they could do this?

The Bridge Between – Breathing and Respiratory Disorders

Normal Respiratory Physiology	What if it Goes Wrong?
Moving O_2 into the blood, and CO_2 out, requires 3 different actions: VENTILATION, PERFUSION, and GAS EXCHANGE.	
VENTILATION is moving air into and out of your lungs.	
You inhale by increasing the size of your chest cavity, creating a low-pressure space that air can fill.	If you couldn't increase the size of the chest cavity, you wouldn't be able to inhale.
The chest cavity can be enlarged by lowering its floor (contracting the diaphragm) or moving its sides outwards using accessory muscles (external intercostal, parasternal, scalene, pectoralis minor, and sternocleidomastoid muscles)	If you could not move these muscles, you would not be able to inhale. Inability to inhale would decrease the amount of O_2 you could bring into your body. Your blood pO_2 would decrease.
When the chest cavity expands, air goes down your airway into your lungs, because that is the only opening it can enter through.	If the airway were blocked, then air wouldn't go into your lungs. If you had another opening into your chest cavity, air might enter through that hole instead of going into your lungs.
The air you inhale fills your airway and then your lungs. The airway is your CONDUCTING ZONE or DEAD SPACE and the alveoli and respiratory bronchioles are the RESPIRATORY ZONE, where O_2 and CO_2 can be exchanged with the blood.	If you took very shallow breaths, you would only inhale enough air to fill your dead space. Without inhaling enough air to reach the respiratory zone, you would have trouble getting enough O_2.
The ALVEOLI of the lungs inflate easily as air enters them, because they are lined with a soapy substance called SURFACTANT.	Without surfactant, it would be too hard for the alveoli to open. You would not be able to inflate your lungs.
To exhale, you relax your diaphragm and accessory muscles. This makes your chest cavity smaller, raising the pressure inside it and pushing air out through your airway. You can also contract your internal intercostal and abdominal muscles to pull your rib cage inward and push your diaphragm upward, for forceful exhalation.	Inability to exhale would reduce your ability to remove CO_2 from the body. Your blood pCO_2 would increase.
The ventilation rate is controlled by two groups of CHEMORECEPTORS that measure the gas and pH levels of your blood and then send impulses to the respiratory neurons in the medulla oblongata.	If you had no chemoreceptors, you would never adjust your breathing to keep blood gases constant. Your pCO_2 and pO_2 would not be regulated.

The CENTRAL CHEMORECEPTORS in your brain respond to acid levels in your cerebrospinal fluid. Because much of the acid in your cerebrospinal fluid is made from CO_2, these sensors respond quickly to increased CO_2 levels in your blood, and cause you to breathe faster and more deeply until the excess CO_2 has been exhaled out of your body. If your blood becomes too acidic for any other reason, that acid will also cause you to breathe faster and more deeply.	If your central chemoreceptors didn't work, you would not respond to high CO_2 levels or excess acid (low pH). You might develop high pCO_2 or low blood pH and not do anything to correct it.
The PERIPHERAL CHEMORECEPTORS in your aorta and carotid arteries respond to CO_2 and pH, but also to O_2 levels. They cause you to breathe when CO_2 is high, pH is low, or O_2 is too low.	If the peripheral chemoreceptors didn't work, you would not change your breathing in response to changing pO_2 levels.
PULMONARY PERFUSION is blood flow through the lungs.	If no blood went through your lungs, you wouldn't be able to carry O_2 from the lungs to the rest of the body.
The right side of the heart pumps blood through the pulmonary trunk and pulmonary arteries to the pulmonary arterioles and capillaries.	If there were trouble with the right heart or these blood vessels were blocked, less blood would reach the lungs to pick up O_2 or drop off CO_2.
The alveoli are covered with PULMONARY CAPILLARIES, bringing blood to pick up O_2 and drop off CO_2.	If the capillaries were damaged, you would not be able to pick up as much O_2 or drop off as much CO_2.
The arterioles that bring blood into these capillaries can open (dilate) and close (constrict). They dilate when there is fresh air in the alveoli, so that the blood is sent to the alveoli that have lots of O_2. When the alveoli contain very little O_2 or contain a lot of CO_2, the pulmonary arterioles constrict. This is called VENTILATION-PERFUSION MATCHING.	If ventilation and perfusion weren't matched, you might waste energy pumping blood to parts of the lung where it would not get any O_2.
After going through the pulmonary capillaries, blood returns to the left side of the heart and is sent to the body.	If there were trouble with the left heart, more blood would stay in the lungs leading to pulmonary edema.
GAS EXCHANGE is when the O_2 in the alveoli diffuses into the blood in the pulmonary capillaries, and CO_2 from the pulmonary capillaries diffuses into the alveolar air and is exhaled.	Diffusion occurs across the alveolar membranes. If some of your alveoli were destroyed, you would not be able to exchange gases as fast.

Test yourself! Breathing and Respiratory Disorders

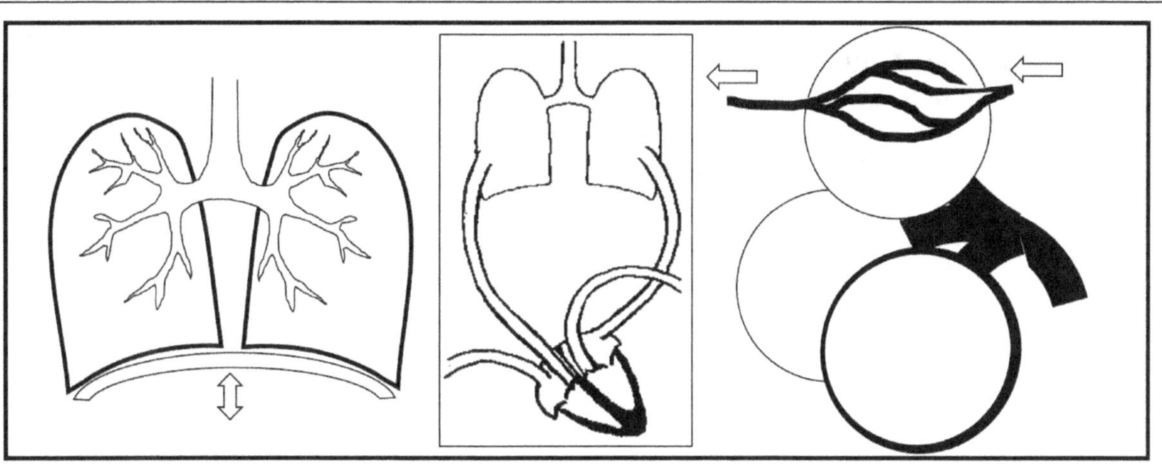

Here are your lungs, attached to your airway. When you move air into and out of the lungs, it is called __________________.

To move air into your lungs you contract your ____________________ to lower the floor of your chest cavity, making more room for air. You can also expand the walls of the chest cavity using your ____________________ muscles.

You need to inhale enough air to fill your ________________ zone and then your ______________ zone. The soapy substance inside the alveoli, __________________, allows your lungs to expand easily as you inhale.

The _____________ side of your heart pumps blood to your lungs through the ______________ trunk and arteries. After the arteries come the P________________ A_______________ and the P__________________ C________________. Perfusion of the lungs is controlled by vasodilation and vasoconstriction. In areas of the lung where there is a lot of O_2 and not very much CO_2, vessels _____________. In areas where there is not much O_2 but a lot of CO_2, vessels ___________. This process is called ventilation-perfusion __________________, and ensures that more blood goes to the areas with fresh air.

Your respiration rate is controlled by two sets of _________________. The C____________ sensors respond to _________ levels in your ____________________ _______. When you accumulate CO_2 in your blood, some of it is converted into ________________ and causes the pH to _____________. These sensors will then cause respiration to ____________________, exhaling more CO_2 and making the pH _____________. The P______________ sensors are located in your _______ and ______________. They stimulate breathing when blood O_2 levels ________________.

Apply it! Breathing and Respiratory Disorders

Mr. S is a fireman who was caught in a collapsing building. He arrived at the emergency room unconscious, with three broken ribs and a sucking chest wound. The EMT had put a dressing over the chest wound. She says, "I don't think we got it fast enough; the lung on this side is collapsed."

A sucking chest wound is an injury that lets air move through a hole in the chest wall into the pleural space outside the lungs. Why would this make the lung collapse?

Doctors inserted a chest tube to remove the air in Mr. S's chest cavity, and his lung reinflated. But later that night, he began to complain of respiratory distress. His pulse oximeter showed a steady decrease, and his lungs sounded wet. "That's what I was afraid of," said one of the nurses. "He inhaled smoke, and now he might be developing ARDS."

In Acute Respiratory Distress Syndrome (ARDS), one problem is that the surfactant in much of the lung tissue is destroyed. Why is this dangerous?

The doctor has Mr. S transferred to the ICU. "We need to measure his pulmonary blood pressure, because it might spike," the doctor says. Why might Mr. S's pulmonary blood pressure go up?

The Bridge Between – Heart Function and Cardiac Disorders

Normal Cardiac Physiology	What if it Goes Wrong?
The heart pumps blood. Each side of the heart has two chambers; an upper ATRIUM that collects venous blood and sends it down to a lower VENTRICLE, which pumps it out of the heart.	If it didn't work, blood wouldn't move around, carrying O_2 and food to your tissues and CO_2 and wastes away from them.
The LEFT HEART takes blood from the lungs (pulmonary circuit) and pumps it to the body (systemic circuit).	If it failed, more blood would stay in the lungs and less would be sent to the body.
The RIGHT HEART takes blood from the body (systemic circuit) and sends it to the lungs (pulmonary circuit).	If it failed, more blood would stay in the systemic veins and less would be sent to the lungs.
During DIASTOLE, the ventricles relax and fill with blood.	If the heart couldn't relax or fill with blood, that blood would stay out in the body and lungs.
During SYSTOLE, the ventricles contract and pump blood out of the heart.	If the heart couldn't contract and pump blood out, less blood would be sent to the body and lungs.
PRELOAD describes the amount of blood entering the heart during diastole, or the pressure caused by filling the heart with blood.	If preload were too small, the heart wouldn't contain much blood to pump out to the body and lungs.
AFTERLOAD is the force the heart must produce during systole to push blood through the vessels in the body and lungs.	If afterload were too high, the heart wouldn't be able to push the blood through the vessels fast enough – and it would be overworked!
The heart muscle needs O_2 and food, just like the rest of the body. It gets them from blood flowing into the coronary arteries. This happens during diastole, when the heart is relaxed.	If blood couldn't flow through coronary arteries, or the diastolic blood pressure was too low (Messerli *et al.* 2006), the heart muscle cells depending on those arteries might not get enough O_2 or food.
The flow of blood between the atria and ventricles is controlled by a set of one-way ATRIOVENTRICULAR (AV) VALVES. During diastole, blood from the body enters the right atrium and flows down through the TRICUSPID VALVE into the right ventricle. Blood from the lungs enters the left atrium and flows down through the BICUSPID or MITRAL VALVE into the left ventricle.	If you didn't have AV valves or they didn't close, blood could flow back and forth between the heart chambers instead of going out to the body and lungs. If an AV valve didn't open properly, blood would stay in the atrium and not enter the ventricle. The atrium would become overloaded with blood and less blood would be sent on out of the heart. This could happen to one side or to both sides of the heart.

During systole, the ventricles contract and push the blood up against the atrioventricular valves. This makes them close, causing the FIRST HEART SOUND – 'lub.' (A for AV valve, it's the FIRST letter).	If an AV valve didn't close properly, blood would go back up into the atrium when the ventricles contract instead of being sent out of the heart to the body or lungs.
When the ventricles contract, blood is forced out of the left ventricle through the AORTIC SEMILUNAR VALVE into the systemic arteries. Blood is forced out of the right ventricle through the PULMONARY SEMILUNAR VALVE into the pulmonary arteries.	If a semilunar valve didn't open properly, less blood would move out of the ventricle to the lungs or body.
When systole ends and diastole starts again, the ventricles are done contracting and relax. Blood is no longer pushed through the semilunar valves and they close. This is the second heart sound, 'dup.' (S for semilunar, S for SECOND sound).	If a semilunar valve didn't close properly, blood would drip back through it into the ventricle during diastole, when the heart is relaxed. The ventricle would be overloaded with blood.
For blood to flow properly, the atria have to contract before the ventricles do. This is controlled by the heart's conduction system.	If the atria and ventricles contracted at the same time, the ventricles would be contracting before they'd been filled with blood. They wouldn't push enough blood out to the lungs or body.
The first part of the heart to fire is the SINOATRIAL (SA) NODE in the right atrium.	If the SA node didn't fire at the proper rate, the heart would not beat at the proper rate.
The SA node will fire automatically, because it has ion channels (HCN channels) that let positively charged ions leak into its cells and depolarize them (Biel *et al.*, 2002).	If the ion channels leaked too much or too little, the heart rate would be changed (Baruscotti *et al.*, 2016).
Heart rate can be adjusted by nerves attached to the SA node.	Without a functioning SA node, the person wouldn't be able to adjust their heart rate as needed.
Sympathetic nerves release norepinephrine. This attaches to beta-1 receptors on the SA node cells, making them depolarize faster.	Without the sympathetic system, norepinephrine, or beta-1 receptors, heart rate would be slow. With too much sympathetic system activity, the heart would beat too fast.
Parasympathetic nerves release acetylcholine, which attaches to muscarinic receptors on the SA node cells and makes them depolarize more slowly (Harvey, 2012).	Without the parasympathetic system, acetylcholine, or muscarinic receptors, heart rate would be fast. With too much parasympathetic system activity, the heart would beat too slowly.

The impulse that began in the SA node spreads across the atria, until they have depolarized. This appears on an EKG trace as the P WAVE. The atria then contract and push blood down into the ventricles.	If the impulse passing across the atria was interfered with, the contraction would be abnormal and less blood might be sent down to the ventricles. The P wave would be altered.
The impulse cannot move directly from the atria to the ventricles. It has to pass through the ATRIOVENTRICULAR (AV) NODE and the BUNDLE OF HIS (or AV bundle). This delays the impulse and gives the ventricles time to fill before they contract. The delay appears on the EKG as a space between the P wave and the QRS complex. It's measured as the PR INTERVAL, between the start of the P wave and the start of the QRS complex.	If the SA node or Bundle of His were damaged, the distance between the P and QRS waves (the PR segment) would become too long and ventricle contraction would be delayed.
After the impulse reaches the ventricles, it runs down the BUNDLE BRANCHES in the ventricular septum and through the PURKINJE FIBERS that take it up the outsides of the ventricles. The ventricular cells receive the impulse and depolarize. That causes the QRS complex on the EKG trace.	If the bundle branches were damaged, the impulse would not run across the ventricles fast enough for all the ventricle cells to contract together. The QRS complex on the EKG would be abnormal.
When the ventricular cells depolarize, they remain depolarized for a while because they have Ca^{2+} channels that allow Ca^{2+} to leak into the cell, keeping it positive. During this PLATEAU period, the cells keep contracting. This is what makes the heartbeat strong enough to push the blood.	If the Ca^{2+} channels didn't let enough calcium in, the cells wouldn't stay depolarized as long and would not have as much time to contract. The heartbeat would be weaker.
After depolarizing, the ventricular cells open their K^+ channels and let K^+ flow out of the cell. This repolarizes them. That appears as the T WAVE on the EKG.	If K^+ levels in the blood were abnormal, the T wave would be abnormal.

Baruscotti, M., Bianco, E., Bucchi, A., & DiFrancesco, D. (2016). Current understanding of the pathophysiological mechanisms responsible for inappropriate sinus tachycardia: role of the If "funny" current. Journal of Interventional Cardiac Electrophysiology: An International Journal of Arrhythmias and Pacing, 46(1), 19–28. https://doi.org/10.1007/s10840-015-0097-y

Biel, M., Schneider, A., & Wahl, C. (2002). Cardiac HCN Channels: Structure, Function, and Modulation. Trends in Cardiovascular Medicine, 12(5), 206–213. https://doi.org/10.1016/S1050-1738(02)00162-7

Harvey, R. D. (2012). Muscarinic receptor agonists and antagonists: effects on cardiovascular function. Handbook of Experimental Pharmacology, (208), 299–316. https://doi.org/10.1007/978-3-642-23274-9_13

Messerli, F. H., Mancia, G., Conti, C. R., Hewkin, A. C., Kupfer, S., Champion, A., ... Pepine, C. J. (2006). Dogma disputed: can aggressively lowering blood pressure in hypertensive patients with coronary artery disease be dangerous? Annals of Internal Medicine, 144(12), 884–893.

Test yourself! Heart Function and Cardiac Disorders

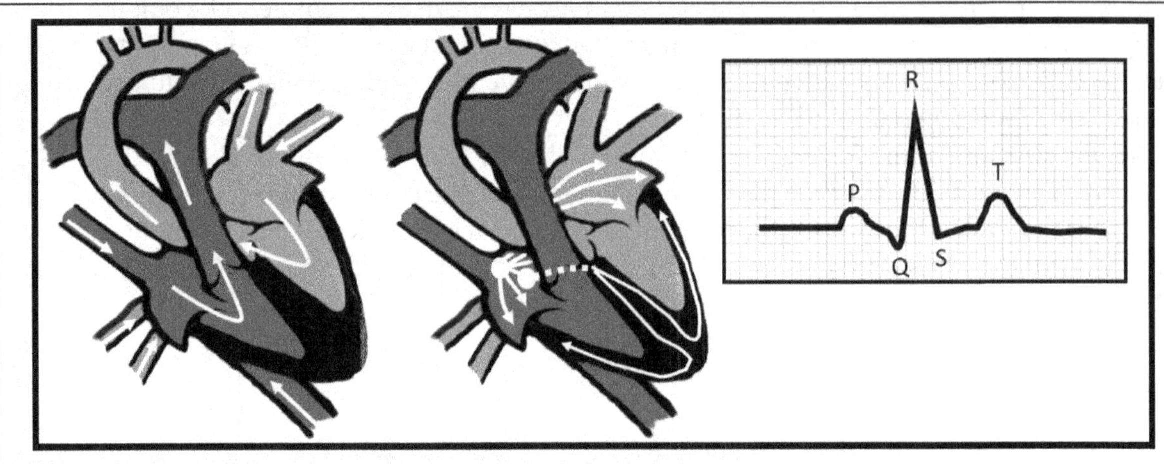

Here's your heart, divided into the right and left sides. Blood from the body enters the _______________, passes through the _______________ valve, and goes into the _______________.
When the heart contracts during _____________, that blood will be pushed out into the _______________ circuit. At the same time, blood from the lungs is entering the _______________ and going down through the _______________ valve into the _______________, which will send it into the _______________ circuit.

When the ventricles contract during _____________, they push blood up against the _____________ and ___________ valves, closing them and causing the first heart sound. The blood is pushed out of the left ventricle through the _______________ valve and pushed out of the right ventricle through the _______________ valve.
When the ventricles stop contracting, these valves snap shut, making the second heart sound.

Contraction starts when the _________ node depolarizes. It depolarizes automatically, but can be speeded up by the _____________________ system or slowed down by the _____________________ system.
The impulse spreads across the ___________, making them depolarize and causing the ____ wave of the EKG. Then the impulse passes through the _____ node and Bundle of _____ into the ventricles. While this is happening, the EKG shows the _________________.
In the ventricles, the impulse flows along the __________ branches and _______________ fibers to make the ventricles depolarize.
When ventricles depolarize, you see the _____________ on the EKG.
Finally, ventricles repolarize again. That causes the _____________ on the EKG.

Apply it! Heart Function and Cardiac Disorders

Ms. P has been feeling weak and tired. She also complains of shortness of breath, and sometimes she wakes up at night with a feeling that she's drowning. Her blood pressure is low, her heart rate is high, and her lungs sound wet. Her pulseox is lower than normal, and you hear a murmur between her first and second heart sounds. The doctor orders a bedside ultrasound, and it reveals that Ms. P's aortic valve isn't opening all the way. Her left ventricle is enlarged.

Has the partly blocked aortic valve affected the heart's preload or afterload?

Why is the left ventricle enlarged?

Why is her blood pressure decreased?

Why is her heart rate increased?

The murmur you heard is the sound of turbulent blood forcing its way through the narrowed valve. Do you hear this sound during diastole or during systole? Why? Why do you hear the sound before the second heart sound?

Does the valve defect explain Ms. P's drowning sensation, or is that a separate problem?

The Bridge Between -- Blood Pressure and its Disorders

Normal Cardiovascular Control of BP	What if it Goes Wrong?
Blood pressure depends on two things: CARDIAC OUTPUT (how much blood your heart pumps) and Peripheral Resistance (also called SYSTEMIC VASCULAR RESISTANCE: basically, how hard it is to push the blood through your vessels).	A change in either CO or PR will alter blood pressure, but because there are two factors controlling blood pressure the body could usually adjust one of them to compensate for changes in the other.
Cardiac output is mL of blood pumped per minute. The most important variables controlling it are: HEART RATE (beats/min) and STROKE VOLUME (mL blood /beat). HR x SV = CO	If heart rate were too low, CO would also be too low. If SV were too low because you didn't have enough blood or your heart didn't pump effectively, then CO would be too low.
SV depends on how much blood enters your heart during diastole (PRELOAD), what percentage of that blood is pumped out during systole (EJECTION FRACTION), and how hard it is for the heart to push the blood out (AFTERLOAD).	If blood couldn't enter your heart effectively or your blood volume was low, then there would not be much blood for the heart to pump on the next beat and CO would be low. If your heart didn't contract strongly enough to move the blood into the arteries, then ejection fraction would be low and so would CO.
BLOOD PRESSURE is the pressure your blood exerts against the walls of your arteries. We measure this by putting a cuff around your arm and seeing how much pressure it takes to compress the artery, but your body measures it using stretch receptors in the walls of your arteries. These receptors are called BARORECEPTORS.	If you didn't have baroreceptors, you would be unable to measure your blood pressure, so you would not be able to regulate it.
The baroreceptors are located in the carotid sinuses and the aortic arch, so they measure systemic blood pressure and the pressure of blood going to your brain.	If something interfered with blood flow in these particular vessels, your body would adjust blood pressure even if the BP was perfectly fine in the rest of the body. If the BP was normal in these vessels, the body would maintain it – even if it was all wrong in other parts of your body.
The baroreceptors measure BP and send the information to the CARDIAC CONTROL and VASOMOTOR centers in the medulla oblongata of your brain. These centers compare the measured BP with the set point.	If these centers weren't working, you would not be able to regulate blood pressure. If the set point changes, you would regulate blood pressure to keep it at the new set point.

If BP is below set point, the cardiac control center can speed up the heart by stimulating SYMPATHETIC NERVES to the heart's pacemaker cells. If BP is above set point, the cardiac control center can slow down the heart by stimulating PARASYMPATHETIC NERVES to the pacemaker cells.	If the cardiac control center didn't function properly, you would be unable to adjust heart rate appropriately to maintain a normal blood pressure. If other parts of your brain activated the sympathetic or parasympathetic systems, they could affect the heart rate even if the cardiac control center wasn't sending specific messages to the heart. For instance, when you're scared your sympathetic system would increase heart rate even if BP is fine.
To raise HR and CO, the sympathetic nerves release norepinephrine which attaches to beta-1 receptors on the pacemaker cells. This causes the heart to beat faster and more strongly.	If your SNS was blocked or the SNS nerves to the heart were damaged or the beta-1 receptors were blocked, you would not be able to effectively increase HR or heart strength. If something else stimulated the sympathetic system, your HR would increase.
To lower HR and CO, the parasympathetic vagus nerve releases acetylcholine which attaches to the muscarinic receptors on the pacemaker cells.	If the vagus nerve was damaged or the muscarinic receptors were blocked, you would have trouble lowering the HR. If something else stimulated the parasympathetic system, your HR would drop.
PERIPHERAL RESISTANCE is how tightly the arterioles are VASOCONSTRICTED. When they are constricted, it is harder to push blood through them; they RESIST the blood, so PR is higher. When they DILATE, they don't resist the blood so much, so PR is lower.	
When arterioles vasoconstrict, less blood can move from the arteries into the capillaries. That means the blood pressure in the arteries increases.	If your arterioles couldn't vasoconstrict, blood would flow through them into all the capillary beds. You don't have enough blood to fill the capillary beds, so your arteries would empty out into them and your blood pressure in the arteries would drop.
When arterioles vasodilate, more blood can move from the arteries into the capillaries. That means the blood pressure in the arteries decreases.	If your arterioles couldn't dilate, you would have trouble supplying blood to the capillary beds in your tissues. All the blood would remain in the arteries, so arterial blood pressure would be high.

If BP is below set point, the vasomotor center can cause arterioles to vasoconstrict, raising the peripheral resistance and the BP. If BP is above set point, the vasomotor center can cause arterioles to vasodilate, decreasing the peripheral resistance and the BP.	If the vasomotor center didn't function properly, you would be unable to vasoconstrict appropriately to maintain a normal blood pressure.
To raise PR, the sympathetic nerves release norepinephrine which attaches to alpha-1 receptors on the arteriolar smooth muscle cells. This causes them to constrict, vasoconstricting the arterioles in the skin, guts, and kidneys.	If your SNS was blocked or the SNS nerves to the heart were damaged or the alpha-1 receptors were blocked, you would not be able to effectively increase PR.
When blood flow to the kidneys decreases, the kidneys activate the renin-ANGIOTENSIN-ALDOSTERONE system (RAAS) to raise blood pressure	If you couldn't activate this pathway, you would have trouble raising blood pressure. If you activated it too much, you would develop high blood pressure.
The juxtaglomerular (or granular) cells sense low blood pressure in the renal arterioles, or react to the sympathetic system. They release renin into the blood.	Without renin, you would not be able to increase blood pressure as effectively.
Renin reacts with the protein angiotensinogen in the blood to form ANGIOTENSIN I. In the lungs, ANGIOTENSIN converting enzyme converts it into ANGIOTENSIN II.	If you didn't have enough angiotensinogen or ANGIOTENSIN converting enzyme, this pathway would not work and you could not raise blood pressure as effectively.
ANGIOTENSIN II helps to increase blood pressure in several ways: - It vasoconstricts, increasing PR - It causes the proximal tubules of the kidneys to reabsorb more sodium - It causes the adrenal cortex to release the hormone ALDOSTERONE	Without ANGIOTENSIN II, you would not be able to raise blood pressure as effectively. With too much of it, you could develop high blood pressure.

ALDOSTERONE causes the kidneys to activate the Na^+/K^+ ATPase, which reabsorbs 3 Na^+ from the urine into the blood, and secretes 2 K^+ from the blood into the urine. Water follows the majority of ions by osmosis – which means it returns to the blood.	If you had too much ALDOSTERONE, you would retain too much Na^+ and water and lose too much K^+ in your urine. If you had too little ALDOSTERONE, you would lose too much Na^+ and water in your urine, and retain too much K^+ in your blood.
If blood volume rises too high, the heart will be over-stretched. The atria will release the hormone ATRIAL NATRIURETIC PEPTIDE. The ventricles will release B-TYPE NATRIURETIC PEPTIDE. Both of these hormones inhibit the SNS and RAAS and cause you to excrete Na+ and water in your urine, decreasing blood volume. All of these actions decrease blood pressure and reduce the workload on the heart.	If you couldn't make these hormones, you probably wouldn't be able to reduce blood volume when the heart was overworked. If you made too much of them, you probably would have trouble increasing blood volume when BP was low – but I couldn't find any cases of imbalances, so this is just speculation.

Test yourself! Blood Pressure and its Disorders

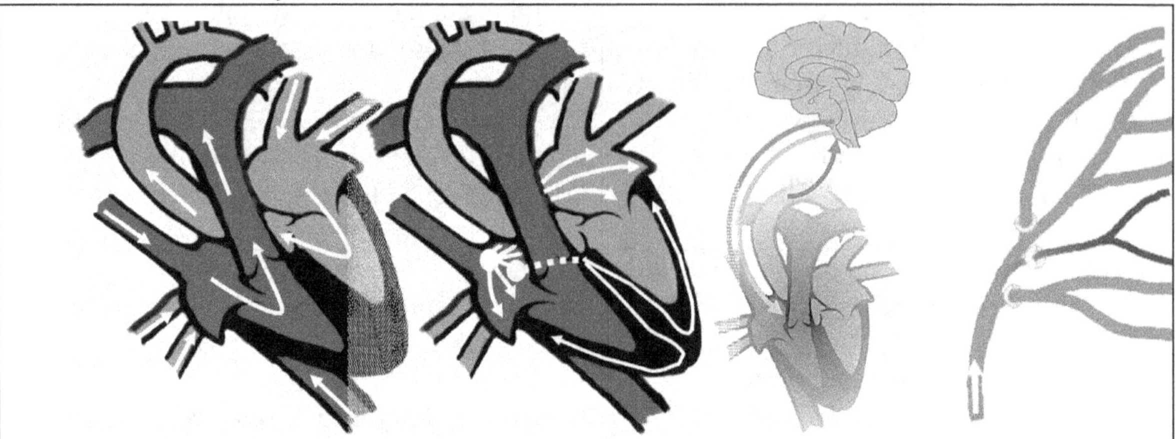

Here's your heart, pumping blood into an artery. The blood presses against the artery walls; this is called the

________________.

The amount of blood the heart pumps into the arteries every minute is the

__________________. It depends on the ______________ and the ________________. If the amount of blood pumped goes down, blood pressure will ____________.

In the artery, the pressure of blood against the artery walls is measured by stretch receptors called

__________________.

They're located in the __________ arteries and the __________.

These receptors send information about the blood pressure to the

__________________ and ______________ centers in the medulla oblongata.

Here's your medulla, getting messages about the blood pressure and comparing it to the

____________.

If BP is too low, the

________________ center in the medulla will tell the heart to ____________, using neurons from the ________________ system.

If blood pressure is too high, the medulla will tell the heart to ________________, using the ________________ system.

The heart isn't the only thing that controls blood pressure. If the blood vessels ____________ and get smaller, they will squeeze on the blood and blood pressure will increase. This is called P______________ R______________.

Here's an arteriole with a sphincter around it. The sphincter can open or close to let blood flow into the capillary bed.

If the sphincter opens, the vessel has V________________.

This will make blood pressure ______. If the sphincter closes, the vessel has V________________ and the blood pressure will ____________.

These sphincters can be controlled by the V________________ center in the medulla oblongata.

If BP is too low, the V________________ center will turn up the ____________ system to make the sphincters ____________. If BP is too high, it will turn this system down, to let the sphincters

__________________.

Apply it! Blood Pressure and its Disorders

A woman having a widespread allergic reaction suffered rapid vasodilation of all her arterioles at once. How will this affect her blood pressure, her medulla oblongata, and her heart rate?

The woman injected herself with an epi pen containing EPINEPHRINE, a sympathetic system stimulant. How would this help her?

When she arrived at the hospital, the doctor noted that her heart rate was very high but her blood pressure was still low. What do you think the woman's peripheral resistance was?

After receiving intravenous fluids, the woman's blood pressure increased. Was this because her cardiac output increased, or her peripheral resistance? Why?

The woman's blood pressure got a little too high after the fluids. What will her medulla oblongata do to bring it down again?

The Bridge Between -- GI function and GI problems

Normal GI Function	What if it Goes Wrong?
The GI tract helps supply the body with nutrients and water.	If the GI tract didn't work, the person would be malnourished and/or dehydrated.
MOTILITY is the movement of food through the GI tract, controlled by rhythmic movements of the smooth muscles in the bowel walls.	If the smooth muscles stopped moving, food would just sit in the bowel. Water would move from the blood into the bowel by osmosis, and the bowel would become distended with food and water.
SECRETION refers to the release of fluid containing mucus, digestive enzymes and acids or bases into the GI tract. DIGESTION is breaking large molecules in the food into smaller molecules that can be passed to the bloodstream.	If secretion or digestion didn't occur, the food would go out in the stools undigested. Water would follow it by osmosis.
ABSORPTION is when the broken-down food molecules are passed to the blood.	If food could not be absorbed, the digested fragments of food would go out in the stools. Water would follow the food by osmosis.
Chewing, swallowing, and salivation are the first events in motility and secretion.	If the muscles involved in swallowing didn't work properly, the person might choke or aspirate food down the trachea into the lungs.
The food mixed with saliva moves down the esophagus through the lower esophageal sphincter to the stomach	If food couldn't pass through the sphincter, it would accumulate in the esophagus. If stomach contents could pass up through the sphincter, the acid in them would irritate the esophagus.
In the stomach, HCl and pepsinogen are secreted. The HCl converts the pepsinogen into pepsin, a protein-digesting enzyme. A layer of mucus protects the stomach's lining from the HCl and pepsin.	Without mucus, the stomach lining could be damaged by the acid and pepsin.
HCl helps you absorb iron from your diet	Without HCl, you might develop iron deficiency (Betesh *et al.*, 2015).
The stomach also secretes INTRINSIC FACTOR, which is needed to absorb Vit B12. Vit B12 is vital for red blood cell production.	Without intrinsic factor, a person would have trouble absorbing Vit. B12. Their red blood cell count would go down.
Stomach secretion is stimulated by the hormone GASTRIN, which is also made by stomach cells.	If there was too much GASTRIN, the stomach would secrete too much acid and pepsin, and they might damage the stomach lining.

As the stomach churns, food is pushed through the pyloric sphincter into the DUODENUM, the first part of the small intestine. The duodenum responds by releasing the hormone GLUCOSE-DEPENDENT INSULINOTROPIC PEPTIDE (GIP) and GLUCAGON-LIKE PEPTIDE 1 (GLP-1), which cause the body to create INSULIN and get ready to take up the food that is being digested and passed to the blood).	I couldn't find information about deficiencies of these in humans… what do you think would happen?
The duodenum also releases the hormone SECRETIN. SECRETIN causes the pancreas to send bicarbonate, an antacid, into the duodenum. This neutralizes the stomach acids. It also inhibits GASTRIN production and allows the stomach to stop working (Fox, 2013).	Without SECRETIN you might not send as much bicarbonate to your duodenum, and that might increase the risk of ulcers (Love, 2008)
The duodenum also secretes the hormone CHOLECYSTOKININ (CCK), which causes the gall bladder to send bile to the duodenum. The bile emulsifies fats, dispersing them in the bowel's contents so that enzymes can effectively digest them (Fox, 2013). CHOLECYSTOKININ also causes the pancreas to send digestive enzymes into the duodenum (Fox, 2013).	Without CCK, bile might not be released into the intestines. It might stay in the gallbladder (Wang *et al.*, 2016). Without pancreatic enzymes, fats, meat fibers (Healthwise, 2012), and carbohydrates (Ladas, Giorgiotis, & Raptis, 1993) wouldn't be digested and would pass out in the stools.
As digestion breaks the food down, the smaller molecules produced are trapped by INTESTINAL VILLI in the small intestine. These are tiny finger-shaped protrusions covered with cells that can grab the food and help finish digesting it. They then pass the food to the lymph vessels or blood vessels inside them.	If a person didn't have enough intestinal villi, the food would not be trapped and absorbed. It would go out in the stools.
Undigested food passes through the ileocecal valve into the large intestine or colon, which contains bacteria. The bacteria break down some of the food, synthesize some vitamins, and protect the colon against the overgrowth of dangerous pathogens. They also produce gas.	If the bacterial community were altered, food breakdown and vitamin synthesis might be altered. Pathogens might be able to grow faster. If the bacteria had too much food to break down, they might produce excess gas. If the large intestine let the bacteria escape, they might infect the body cavity or enter the blood.

Cells lining the large intestine absorb ions into the blood, and water follows the ions by osmosis	If the large intestine couldn't absorb ions, the ions and the water would be lost in the stools. The person would become dehydrated.
Undigested food will be collected in the sigmoid colon and passed to the rectum. It is released through the anus.	If food couldn't be released in stools, it would accumulate and distend the rectum and colon.

Betesh, A. L., Santa Ana, C. A., Cole, J. A., & Fordtran, J. S. (2015). Is achlorhydria a cause of iron deficiency anemia? The American Journal of Clinical Nutrition, 102(1), 9–19. https://doi.org/10.3945/ajcn.114.097394

Fox, S.I. (2013). Human Physiology, 13th ed. McGraw-Hill.

Healthwise Staff. (2012, March 7). Stool Analysis: Healthwise Medical Information on eMedicineHealth. Retrieved March 28, 2017, from http://www.emedicinehealth.com/stool_analysis-health/article_em.htm

Ladas, S. D., Giorgiotis, K., & Raptis, S. A. (1993). Complex carbohydrate malabsorption in exocrine pancreatic insufficiency. Gut, 34(7), 984–987.

Love, J. W. (2008). Peptic ulceration may be a hormonal deficiency disease. *Medical Hypotheses, 70*(6), 1103–1107. https://doi.org/10.1016/j.mehy.2007.12.011

Wang, H. H., Liu, M., Portincasa, P., Tso, P., & Wang, D. Q.-H. (2016). Lack of endogenous CHOLECYSTOKININ promotes cholelithogenesis in mice. Neurogastroenterology and Motility : The Official Journal of the European Gastrointestinal Motility Society, 28(3), 364–375. https://doi.org/10.1111/nmo.12734

Test Yourself! GI function and GI problems

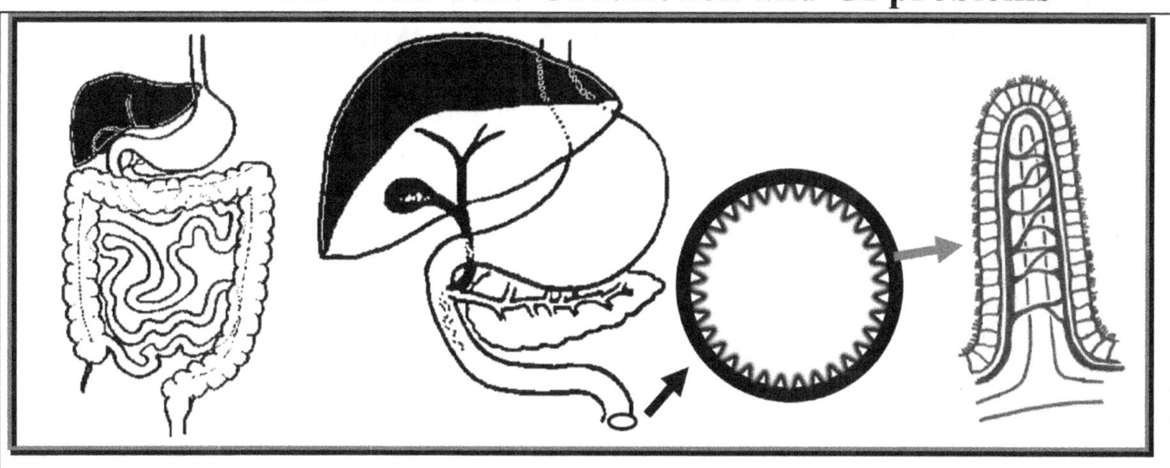

Here's your GI tract, ready to carry out its four functions:

_______________,

_______________,

_______________, and

_______________.

Swallowing moves food into the _______________. The food passes through the _______________ _______________ sphincter into the stomach, where it is mixed with HCl and _______________.
In your stomach, the HCl converts the _______________ into _______________, which begins the digestion of _______________.
HCl is also needed for absorption of _______.
The stomach is protected from the HCl by a layer of _______.
Vit B12 is absorbed using _______________, which is also produced by the stomach.
As long as food is in the stomach, stomach cells will release the hormone _______________, which stimulates more stomach secretion.

Here's the beginning of your small intestine, where the food will go next.

When food finally leaves the stomach, it will go through the _______________ into the _______________.
Three digestive hormones are released: _______ causes the body to make INSULIN, _______________ turns off stomach secretion and makes the _______________ release bicarbonate (antacid), and _______________ makes the gall bladder release _______ and the _______________ release digestive enzymes.

Here's a section of your small intestine showing the finger-like _______________.
Their job is to _______________ the food from the intestinal contents and pass it to the blood or lymph. Food you haven't digested will move through the _______________ valve into the _______, where bacteria break some of it down and produce _______. This region of the intestine also absorbs _______________ and _______________ into the blood.
Undigested food passes into the _______________ and out the _______________.

The Bridge Between – Liver Function and Liver Failure

Normal Liver Physiology	What if it Goes Wrong?
The liver receives blood from all the digestive system organs through the HEPATIC PORTAL VEIN. It then filters the blood. Among its many functions, the liver:	If blood couldn't flow through the liver, the pressure in the hepatic portal vein and the veins that drain into it from the organs will increase. The person could develop varicose veins inside their abdomen.
Deals with TOXINS and HORMONES:	
Breaks down alcohol The liver does this using enzymes, which it can produce in different quantities depending on how much they are used.	If the liver couldn't do this, alcohol would have a stronger effect on the person (Cederbaum, 2012).
Converts toxins (including many meds) into water-soluble forms that can be removed from the body via the urine	If the liver couldn't convert toxins, they might build up in the body and poison the person. A normal dose of medication might give this person an overdose (Periáñez-Párraga *et al.*, 2012).
Breaks down many hormones, stopping their function. ALDOSTERONE is one example.	If ALDOSTERONE weren't broken down it would keep functioning, moving Na^+ and water into the blood and K^+ into the urine. Blood volume would increase and blood K^+ would decrease.
Removes bilirubin from the blood and coverts it into bile, which is used to emulsify fats in the GI tract	If bile weren't made, bilirubin would build up in the blood and tissues causing jaundice. The lack of bile in the GI tract would make it difficult to digest fats, which would be lost in the stools.
Converts ammonia to urea	If ammonia builds up in the blood, it could be toxic to the central nervous system.
Synthesizes BLOOD PROTEINS	
Synthesizes albumin, the primary protein that maintains blood osmolarity	Without albumin, blood osmolarity would decrease. This means that water would move from the blood into the cells, causing cell swelling.
Synthesizes clotting proteins – both procoagulation and anticoagulation factors.	Without these the person would be at risk for bruising and bleeding, or for increased clotting. They wouldn't be able to balance their clotting system.

Converts nutrients and maintains normal blood levels of them	
Sugars are stored in the liver as GLYCOGEN; when the body needs more sugar, the liver breaks down the glycogen and releases GLUCOSE into the blood. If you only ate fat or protein, the liver converts some of it to glucose to keep your blood glucose levels stable. If you ate excess carbohydrates, the liver would convert some of them to fats for storage.	Without this function, blood glucose would be less stable
If you only eat fat and protein, or if you are fasting and using your stored fat and protein, the liver converts some of them into ketoacids which the brain can use for fuel.	This is a puzzler! Morisco *et al.* (2013) found MORE ketones in the breath of people with liver cirrhosis. Apparently, the liver maintains its ability to make ketones even when its other functions have decreased.
The liver converts fats you ate into LIPOPROTEINS, which travel through the blood carrying the fat to cells that need it.	When this doesn't happen, the unprocessed fat could build up in the liver. That could cause fatty liver (Satyanarayana, 2014).

Cederbaum, A. I. (2012). ALCOHOL METABOLISM. Clinics in Liver Disease, 16(4), 667–685. https://doi.org/10.1016/j.cld.2012.08.002

Morisco, F., Aprea, E., Lembo, V., Fogliano, V., Vitaglione, P., Mazzone, G., … Biasioli, F. (2013). Rapid "Breath-Print" of Liver Cirrhosis by Proton Transfer Reaction Time-of-Flight Mass Spectrometry. A Pilot Study. PLOS ONE, 8(4), e59658. https://doi.org/10.1371/journal.pone.0059658

Periáñez-Párraga, L., Martínez-López, I., Ventayol-Bosch, P., Puigventós-Latorre, F., & Delgado-Sánchez, O. (2012). Drug dosage recommendations in patients with chronic liver disease. Rev Esp Enferm Dig, 104(4), 165–184.

Satyanarayana, U. (2014). Biochemistry. Elsevier Health Sciences.

Test yourself! Liver Function and Liver Failure

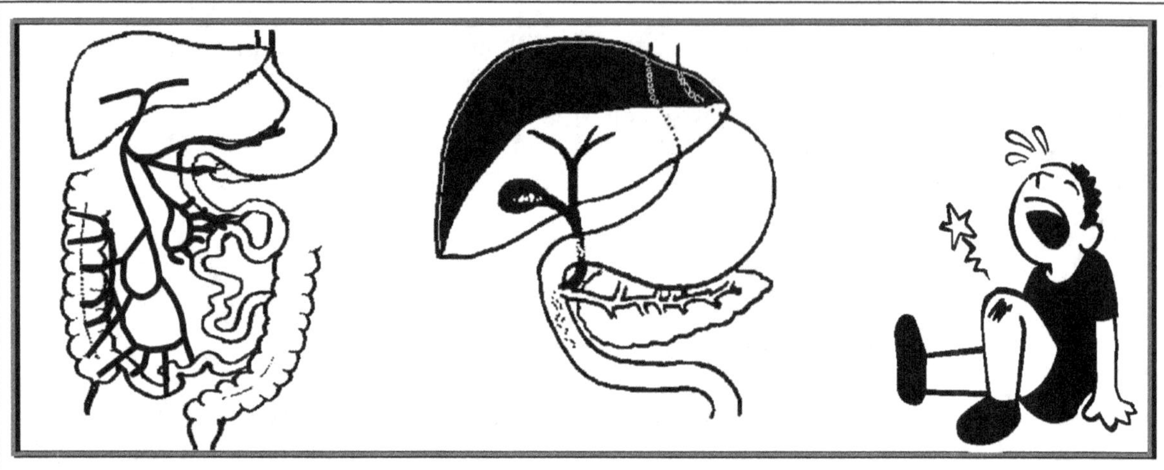

Here's your liver, getting blood from the GI organs through the

____

____

If you just ate a lot of sugar, the liver will store it as

__________________.

But if you haven't eaten, the liver will break the

______________ **down and release glucose into your blood.**

If you only ate fats and proteins, the liver will convert some of them into

______________ **to keep your blood levels stable.**

It will also make some of the fats and proteins into

__________________.

TOXINS! The liver will break these down into

______________-**soluble forms that can be excreted in your urine.**

The liver removes bilirubin from the blood and makes it into

____________, **which is stored in the gall bladder and sent to the intestines where it helps**

________________**fats.**

The liver converts ammonia into __________.

The liver also breaks down hormones like

__________________.

Without the liver, the ____________ **pump in the kidneys would keep running.**

Your liver also produces

____

and

____

factors. Without these you might bleed too much. – or too little.

Another blood protein the liver produces is

__________________,

which maintains the blood osmolarity.

The liver packages fats into

__________________,

which carry them to the cells.

Images of pills and crying boy from Microsoft clip art, 2013

Apply it! Liver Function and Liver Failure

Mr. X has been drinking for years, and his doctor tells him he has alcoholic liver disease and fat malabsorption. Mr. X says this is nonsense, because his problem is booze – not fat! He shows you how thin his arms and legs are. "Not an ounce of fat on 'em!" he says. "That's not what I mean," the doctor says. "I mean you're not digesting the fat you eat." Why can't Mr. X digest fat properly?

Mr. X has yellow skin and the whites of his eyes are yellow as well. What caused this?

When you look at Mr. X's arms you notice a lot of bruises and some scabs. He says "I have thin skin, I bruise myself all the time." How could his liver disease be related to this?

The doctor has ordered some blood tests on Mr. X – Potassium (K^+), ammonia, and blood osmolarity. What do you think they will show?

The Bridge Between – Pancreas Function and Pancreatic Disorders

Normal Pancreas Physiology	What if it Goes Wrong?
Your pancreas is two glands in one – the EXOCRINE pancreas and the ENDOCRINE pancreas	
The <u>ex</u>ocrine pancreas is made up of lots of tiny hollow lobules. They produce digestive enzymes and bicarbonate, which drain out the pancreatic duct into your duodenum. There, they neutralize stomach acids and help you digest your food.	Without pancreatic enzymes, fats, meat fibers (Healthwise, 2012), and carbohydrates (Ladas, Giorgiotis, & Raptis, 1993) wouldn't be digested and would pass out in the stools.
The **<u>endo</u>crine pancreas** is made of tiny clusters of cells called the **Islets of Langerhans** or **Pancreatic Islets.** These do not have any ducts, but instead release their secretions directly into the blood.	
INSULIN is released from the **beta cells** of the pancreatic islets when blood glucose is high. It allows cells to pick up glucose from the blood. That glucose can be burned to make ATP, or it can be stored as glycogen.	Without INSULIN, the glucose could not enter your cells and would stay in your blood. With too much INSULIN, your cells would take up so much glucose that the glucose levels in your blood might drop too low to supply your brain's needs.
GLUCAGON is released from the **alpha cells** of the pancreatic islets when blood glucose levels are low (when your GLUcose is GONe). It causes liver cells that have stored sugar as glycogen to release it into the blood as glucose. It also makes cells break down fats and protein and release them into the blood as free fatty acids and amino acids. Some of the free fatty acids and amino acids are converted into ketoacids by the liver.	With too much GLUCAGON, your blood glucose levels and free fatty acid levels would rise. Without GLUCAGON, your blood glucose levels would drop (Fanelli *et al.*, 2006).

Fanelli, C. G., Porcellati, F., Rossetti, P., & Bolli, G. B. (2006). Glucagon: the effects of its excess and deficiency on INSULIN action. Nutrition, Metabolism, and Cardiovascular Diseases: NMCD, 16 Suppl 1, S28-34. https://doi.org/10.1016/j.numecd.2005.10.018

Healthwise Staff. (2012, March 7). Stool Analysis: Healthwise Medical Information on eMedicineHealth. Retrieved March 28, 2017, from http://www.emedicinehealth.com/stool_analysis-health/article_em.htm

Ladas, S. D., Giorgiotis, K., & Raptis, S. A. (1993). Complex carbohydrate malabsorption in exocrine pancreatic insufficiency. Gut, 34(7), 984–987.

Test yourself! Pancreas Function and Pancreatic Disorders

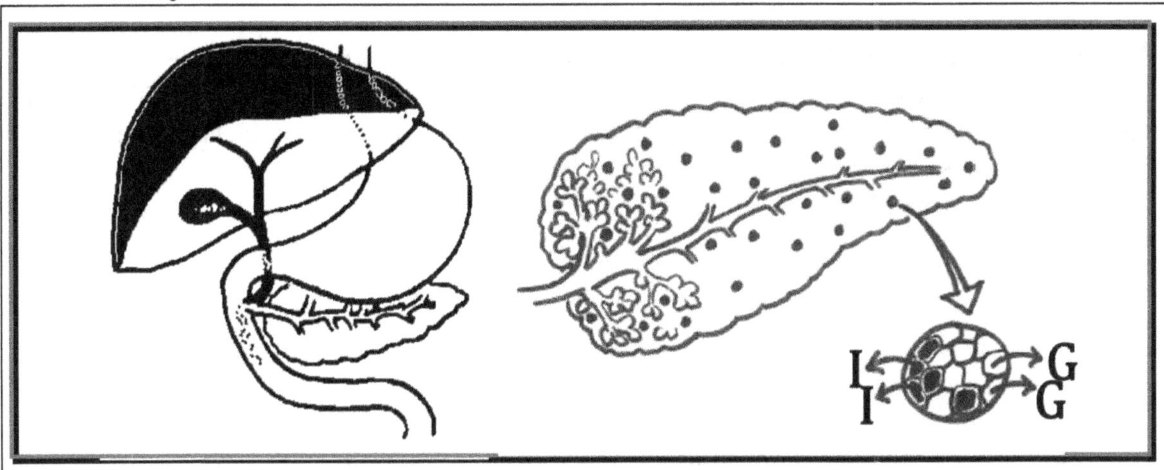

Here's your pancreas, right below your stomach. The ________________ pancreas sends ___________ and _________ through the duct to your duodenum, where they help digest food and ___________________ acid.

The _____________ pancreas is not attached to the pancreatic duct. It is made up of the ___________________________, which secrete hormones into the blood.

When you have high blood sugar levels, the ___________ cells secrete ________________, which allows your cells to ___________________ the sugar from your blood and store it as ________________.

When your blood glucose levels are low, the _______ cells secrete ______________, which makes your cells break down food and release it into the blood.

When you're hungry, your cells break stored ________________ into glucose and release it. They break stored fats into ___________________ and proteins into ___________________.

Your liver will convert some of these into ___________________.

Blood pH will ____________ because of all the ___________.

Apply it! Pancreas Function and Pancreatic Disorders

A child has diabetes mellitus and cannot make INSULIN, but he can make
GLUCAGON. He comes into hospital with weight loss, high blood glucose, high levels of
amino acids and free fatty acids in his blood, high levels of ketones, heavy breathing, and
dehydrated cells.
How did his lack of INSULIN contribute to his high blood glucose?

How did his GLUCAGON contribute to his high blood glucose?

Which of the two hormones is responsible for his high amino acid, free fatty acid, and
ketoacid levels? How?

Which of the two hormones is most responsible for his weight loss? How?

Why are his cells becoming dehydrated? How do you think he will try to compensate for
that?

The Bridge Between – Thyroid Function and Thyroid Disorders

Normal Thyroid Physiology	What if it Goes Wrong?
The thyroid gland produces two hormones: TRIIODOTHYRONINE (T3) and TETRAIODOTHYRONINE (T4 or THYROXIN). Both contain iodine. T3 is the active form of the hormone; T4 can be quickly converted to T3 in the tissues just by removing one iodine from it.	If you didn't have any iodine in your diet, you wouldn't be able to make thyroid hormones.
Thyroid hormone secretion is controlled by the hypothalamus. When your T3 and T4 levels are too low, or you're cold, or you are really well-fed (Nilni, 2010), the hypothalamus secretes THYROTROPIN RELEASING HORMONE (TRH).	Without TRH, you wouldn't create enough T3 or T4. With too much TRH, you'd create too much T3 and T4.
The TRH from the hypothalamus travels to the anterior pituitary, where it tells the pituitary cells to release THYROTROPIN, or THYROID STIMULATING HORMONE (TSH). TSH enters the blood and travels to the thyroid, telling the thyroid to make T3 and T4.	Without TSH, you wouldn't create enough T3 or T4. With too much TSH, you'd create too much T3 and T4.
When your thyroid responds and creates the T3 and T4, the hypothalamus and anterior pituitary detect them in the blood. That causes the hypothalamus to stop making TRH and the anterior pituitary to stop making TSH.	If your thyroid didn't make enough T3 and T4, the hypothalamus and anterior pituitary would keep making TRH and TSH. If you had excess T3 and T4, the levels of TRH and TSH would decrease.
T3 affects cell metabolism, increasing aerobic respiration and the number of mitochondria. It raises metabolic rates and is vital for proper growth and development.	With low levels of T3, brain development and growth would be affected. Aerobic respiration would decrease and there would be less ATP for muscle and nervous function. Food would not be burned for energy, leading to weight gain and low body temperature. With too much T3, too much food would be burned for ATP and muscle and nerves would be hyperactive. Body temperature would increase and weight would decrease..

[1] Nillni, E. A. (2010). Regulation of the Hypothalamic Thyrotropin Releasing Hormone (TRH) Neuron by Neuronal and Peripheral Inputs. *Frontiers in Neuroendocrinology*, *31*(2), 134–156. https://doi.org/10.1016/j.yfrne.2010.01.001

Test Yourself! Thyroid Function and Thyroid Disorders

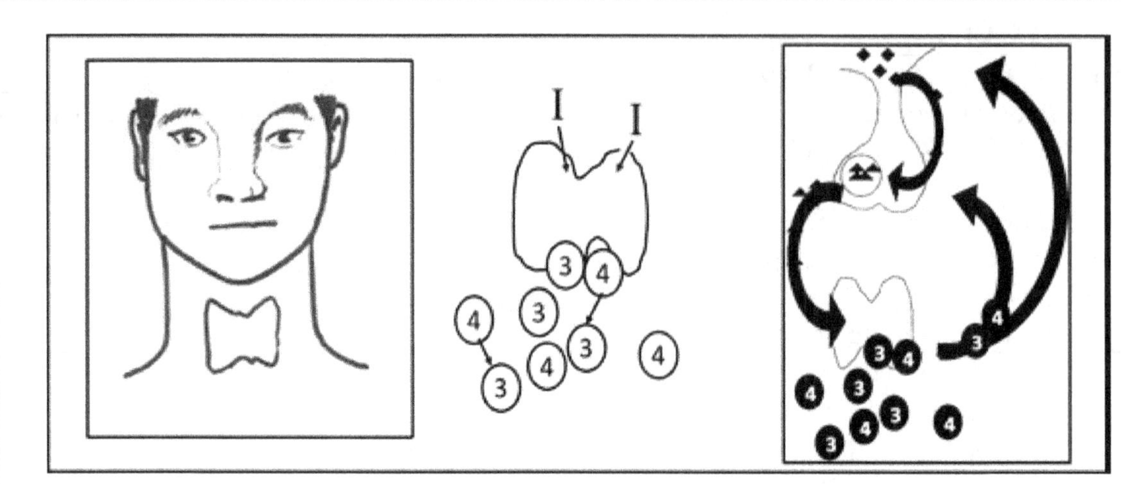

Here's your thyroid, right below your adam's apple. The thyroid releases

____

and

____

into your blood.
The active hormone is

______________________,

and it ____________ your metabolic rate by stimulating __________ respiration. You make __________ ATP, leading to increased __________ and __________ firing and weight _________.
The other hormone,

______________________,

is converted into

____

when your tissues need it.

Your thyroid is controlled by the

______________________, a region of your brain that secretes

____

Releasing Hormone when it is stimulated by cold or __________ levels of

____

and

______________________.

The ______________________ Releasing Hormone goes to your

______________________,

which then releases

______________________, or ______________________ Stimulating Hormone.

The ______________________ Stimulating Hormone travels through the blood to the ____________, stimulating it to release

____

and ______________________.

The hypothalamus and

____

continue secreting their Releasing and Stimulating hormones until they detect normal levels of

____

and

______________________ in the blood.

The Bridge Between – Adrenal Cortex Function and Adrenal Disorders

Normal Adrenal Cortex Physiology	What if it Goes Wrong?
The adrenal cortex is the outer layer of the adrenal glands. It produces many hormones, including ALDOSTERONE,CORTISOL, and TESTOSTERONE. They are all steroid hormones, made from cholesterol.	If you weren't able to make one of these hormones, your adrenal cortex might use the cholesterol to make more of the other hormones.
MINERALOCORTICOIDS are adrenal cortex hormones that control electrolytes. ALDOSTERONE is the best-known of these. Its secretion is mainly controlled by the RAAS pathway. It activates the renal Na^+/K^+ pump, moving Na^+ and water from the urine into the blood and K^+ from the blood into the urine. ALDOSTERONE will also be released if blood K^+ levels are too high. It will activate the pump and move that excess K^+ out of the blood into the urine. When K^+ levels are low, less ALDOSTERONE will be released. That way the body will be able to retain the K^+.	If the RAAS pathway were overactive, you'd make too much ALDOSTERONE. Too much ALDOSTERONE would cause you to reabsorb too much Na^+ and water, increasing blood volume, and you would lose too much K^+ in the urine, leading to low blood K^+. Without ALDOSTERONE, you would not be able to retain Na^+ and water and you would not be able to get rid of excess K^+. Your blood volume would decrease, and blood K+ would increase.
GLUCOCORTICOIDS are hormones from the adrenal cortex that regulate blood glucose.CORTISOL is the best-known of these. Its secretion is controlled by the hypothalamus. When yourCORTISOL levels are too low, or you're stressed, the hypothalamus secretes CORTICOTROPIN RELEASING HORMONE (CRH).	Without CRH, you wouldn't create enoughCORTISOL. With too much CRH, you'd create too muchCORTISOL.
The CRH from the hypothalamus travels to the anterior pituitary, where it tells the pituitary cells to release CORTICOTROPIN, or ADRENAL CORTICOTROPHIC HORMONE (ACTH). ACTH enters the blood and travels to the adrenal cortex, telling it to makeCORTISOL.	Without ACTH, you wouldn't create enoughCORTISOL. With too much ACTH, you'd create too muchCORTISOL.

When your adrenal cortex responds and creates theCORTISOL, the hypothalamus and anterior pituitary detect it in the blood. That causes the hypothalamus to stop making CRH and the anterior pituitary to stop making ACTH.	If your adrenal cortex didn't make enoughCORTISOL, the hypothalamus and anterior pituitary would keep making CRH and ACTH. If you had excessCORTISOL, the levels of CRH and ACTH would decrease.
Cortisol is also called the stress hormone. It makes your cells release stored glucose and break down fat and muscle. Some of these compounds are converted to glucose, raising your blood glucose levels. Cortisol also strengthens your response to the sympathetic system. It can also decrease immune system function and the creation of fibroblasts, cells involved in skin repair and scar tissue.	With low levels ofCORTISOL, you wouldn't be able to raise blood glucose when your cells needed it to help deal with stress. Your blood pressure might decrease. With high levels ofCORTISOL, your blood glucose might go too high. With long periods of highCORTISOL, your muscles might become weak as protein breaks down. Fat would move from your arms and legs to your head, neck, and trunk. Your immune system would be suppressed and your skin might become thin.
ADRENAL ANDROGENS are hormones from the adrenal that cause the development of masculine characteristics. TESTOSTERONE is the best-known of these. Testosterone production from the adrenal cortex can affect the development of external sexual characteristics in fetuses and contribute to the beginning stages of puberty, the adrenarche.	A woman with too much TESTOSTERONE might have excessive pubic and axillary hair growth. A fetus with too much adrenal androgen might become virilized, or masculinized. A fetus with too little adrenal androgen might develop feminized genitalia.

Test Yourself! Adrenal Cortex Function and Adrenal Disorders

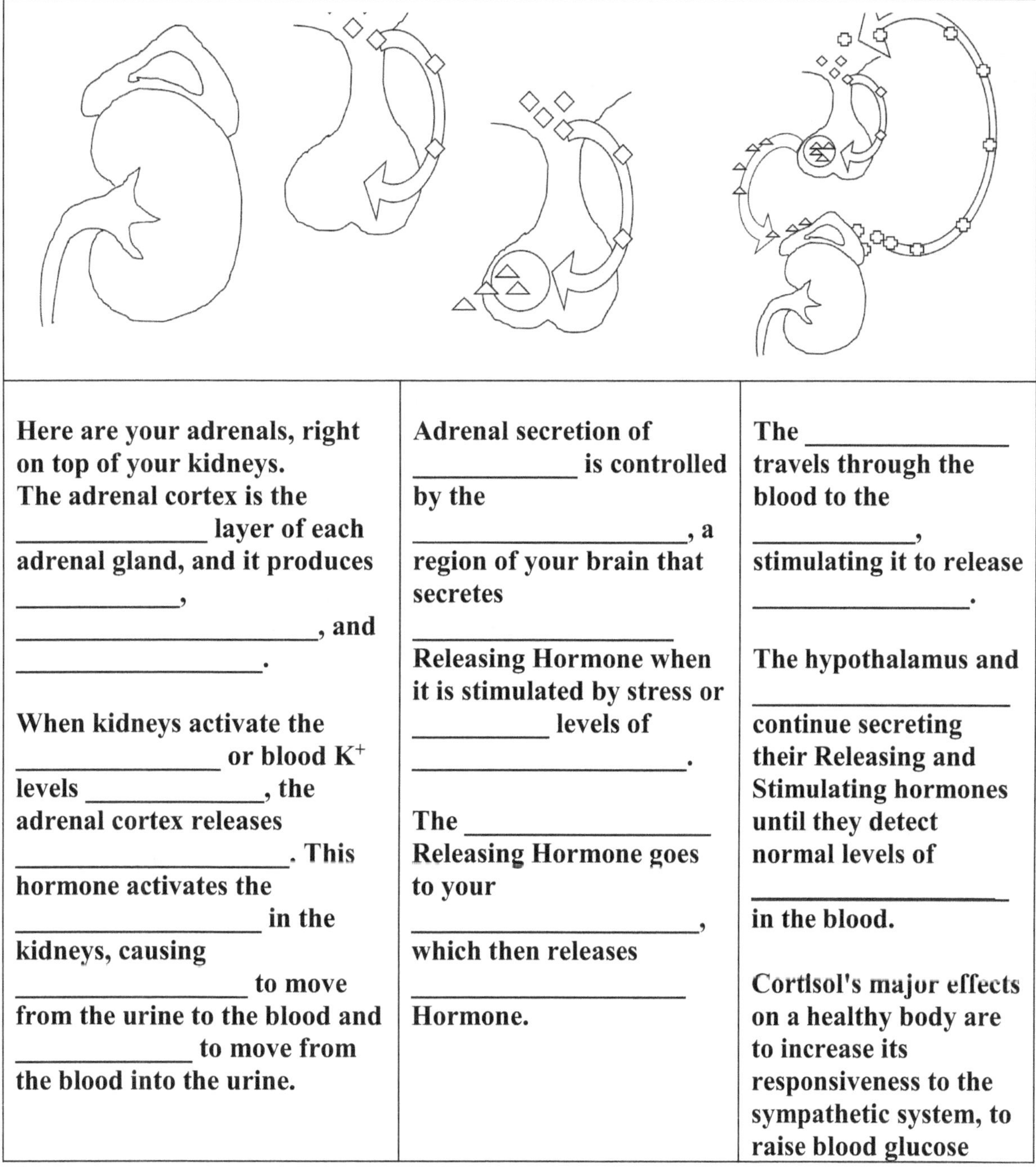

Here are your adrenals, right on top of your kidneys. The adrenal cortex is the ______________ layer of each adrenal gland, and it produces ______________, ______________________, and ______________________.

When kidneys activate the ______________ or blood K^+ levels ______________, the adrenal cortex releases ______________________. This hormone activates the ______________________ in the kidneys, causing ______________________ to move from the urine to the blood and ______________ to move from the blood into the urine.

Adrenal secretion of ______________ is controlled by the ______________________, a region of your brain that secretes ______________________ Releasing Hormone when it is stimulated by stress or ______________ levels of ______________________.

The ______________________ Releasing Hormone goes to your ______________________, which then releases ______________________ Hormone.

The ______________________ travels through the blood to the ______________, stimulating it to release ______________________.

The hypothalamus and ______________________ continue secreting their Releasing and Stimulating hormones until they detect normal levels of ______________________ in the blood.

Cortisol's major effects on a healthy body are to increase its responsiveness to the sympathetic system, to raise blood glucose

Apply it! Adrenal Cortex Function and Adrenal Disorders

A child's parents have brought him in to the clinic because they are afraid he has diabetes mellitus. "He's always urinating, and that's a sign," says his mom. "And he's thirsty all the time."

The doctor asks whether the boy is hungry or losing weight. "He isn't losing weight, but we can't keep him away from the chips and sweets," says his mom. "If we won't let him have snacks, he eats salt right out of the salt shaker!"

The doctor takes the boy's vital signs and observes that his blood pressure is low, and his heart rate is elevated. A blood glucose test shows that the boy's blood glucose is low. "I don't think it's diabetes," the doctor says. "I think his adrenal cortex isn't working right."

Which adrenal cortex hormone is related to blood pressure and salt levels? How is it related to them? Do you think this boy has too much of that hormone, or too little?

Which adrenal cortex hormone is related to blood glucose levels? How is it related to them? Do you think this boy has too much of that hormone, or too little?

The doctor has ordered blood tests for $[K^+]$, ACTH, andCORTISOL. Why are these tests relevant, and what do you expect their values to be? (high, normal, or low)

The tests show thatCORTISOL levels are low, but ACTH is high. Does this indicate that there is a problem with the boy's anterior pituitary as well as his adrenal cortex?

The Bridge Between – Parathyroid Function and Parathyroid Disorders

Normal Parathyroid Physiology	What if it Goes Wrong?
The **parathyroid** glands secrete PARATHYROID HORMONE (PTH) when blood calcium levels are too low.	If blood calcium stayed low, your parathyroids would keep secreting PTH.
PARATHYROID HORMONE helps you absorb calcium from your diet – IF you also have activated VITAMIN D3. PTH also helps you reabsorb calcium from your urine.	Without PARATHYROID HORMONE or activated VITAMIN D3, you wouldn't effectively absorb the calcium. It would be lost in your stools and urine.
VITAMIN D3 is a fat-soluble vitamin that you can get from your diet, IF you can digest fats. You also make it in your skin when you are exposed to UV light. Whether you eat it or make it, the VITAMIN D3 must be activated by your kidneys.	If you didn't make or take in enough VITAMIN D3, or couldn't absorb it or activate it in the kidneys, you would have low VITAMIN D3 and calcium levels.
When PARATHYROID HORMONE is first released, it stimulates the **osteoblasts**, the bone-building cells. But that changes if the PARATHYROID HORMONE levels stay high (Aslan *et al.*, 2012).	Giving someone a single injection of PARATHYROID HORMONE every day will strengthen their bones! It's a treatment for osteoporosis (Quattrocchi & Kourlas, 2004).
If PARATHYROID HORMONE levels **stay** high, they cause different cells, your **osteoclasts**, to release calcium from the bones into the blood.	Without sustained release of PARATHYROID HORMONE, the bones wouldn't release calcium into the blood and blood calcium levels might remain too low. With too much PARATHYROID HORMONE, the bones would release too much calcium into the blood, and the blood calcium might become too high. The bones might become weak and easy to break.

Aslan, D., Andersen, M. D., Gede, L. B., de Franca, T. K., Jørgensen, S. R., Schwarz, P., & Jørgensen, N. R. (2012). Mechanisms for the bone anabolic effect of PARATHYROID HORMONE treatment in humans. *Scandinavian Journal of Clinical and Laboratory Investigation*, *72*(1), 14–22.

Quattrocchi, E., & Kourlas, H. (2004). Teriparatide: a review. *Clinical Therapeutics*, *26*(6), 841–854.

Test yourself! Parathyroid Function and Parathyroid Disorders

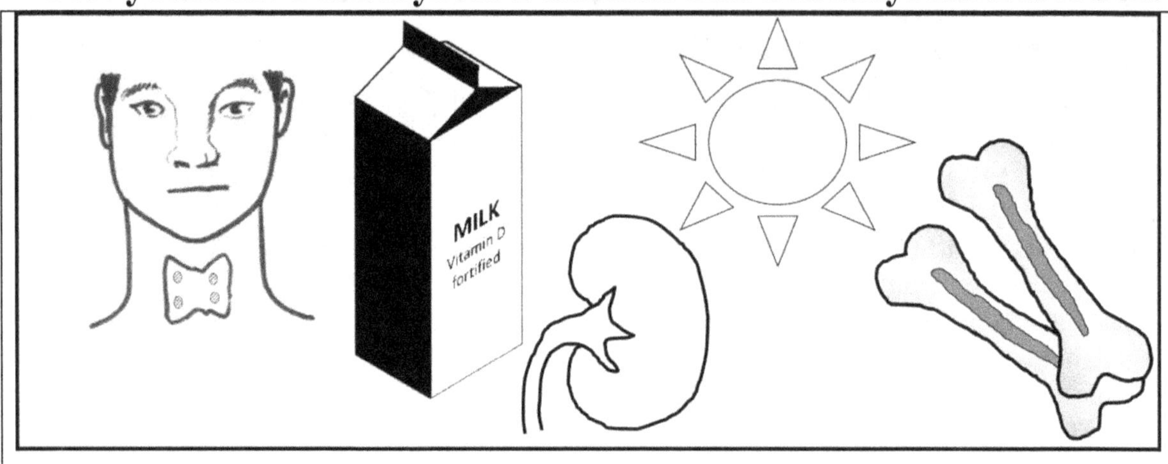

Here are your parathyroids, shown in green. They are attached to the back of your thyroid.

When blood ___________ levels are too low, they secrete

____

___________________.

This hormone helps you bring blood ___________ levels back up to normal.

___________________helps you absorb _____________ from your diet.

It also helps you reabsorb it from your _________ into your ___________.

When blood ____________ levels return to normal, the parathyroids will _________ secreting ___________________.

When they first begin secreting ____________, the parathyroids stimulate

___________________ cells. The ___________ you're absorbing will be deposited in your

_______________.

If ________________ levels remain high for too long, though, the

___________________ cells will be stimulated and they will start to release ___________ from your _________ into the blood.

Bone image from Pixabay, https://pixabay.com/en/bone-dog-skeleton-157272/ : public domain

The Bridge Between – Kidney Function and Renal Disorders

Normal Kidney Physiology	What if it Goes Wrong?
Your kidneys' main job is to regulate the volume and composition of your blood.	Without kidney function wastes would build up in your blood, and you would not be able to control blood volume or composition.
Each of your kidney is made up of microscopic renal tubules, or NEPHRONS. Each nephron filters some of your blood and forms some urine. The urine is then collected in the renal pelvis, which drains into the ureters and bladder.	The fewer nephrons you have, the less effective your kidneys will be at cleaning the blood. If your ureters were blocked, the kidneys would fill up and be unable to produce more urine.
The first step in kidney function is FILTRATION of the blood that enters your kidneys through the renal artery.	If the renal artery is blocked, renal filtration will decrease.
The renal artery branches inside the kidney, finally forming tiny AFFERENT ARTERIOLES.	If the afferent arterioles constrict or are blocked, renal filtration will decrease.
The afferent arterioles all end in tiny capillary beds called GLOMERULI, located in the outer layer of the kidney (the RENAL CORTEX). About 125 mL of blood is filtered through these capillaries every minute. This is the GLOMERULAR FILTRATION RATE or GFR.	Damage to the glomeruli will affect what filters out into the urine and how fast blood is filtered. If the GLOMERULAR FILTRATION RATE drops too low, wastes will begin to build up in the blood.
The walls of the glomerular capillaries let water and most solutes through into the urine, but they stop cells and most proteins. Those stay in the blood and leave the kidneys through the EFFERENT ARTERIOLES and the renal vein.	If the glomeruli are damaged, proteins and cells may appear in the urine.
The fluid that has filtered across your glomeruli is called ULTRAFILTRATE. Each glomerulus sends its ultrafiltrate into its nephron.	If some of the glomeruli are partly blocked, the nephrons attached to them will get less ultrafiltrate.
The nephron begins with an enlarged area called BOWMAN'S CAPSULE. This segment folds around the glomerulus, catching all the ultrafiltrate that is leaking across the glomerular capillaries.	If Bowman's capsule is blocked (for instance, by the build-up of scar tissue), then filtration will decrease.
The ultrafiltrate flows from Bowman's capsule into the first part of the nephron, the PROXIMAL CONVOLUTED TUBULE (PCT). ('Proximal' because it is closest to the glomerulus; 'convoluted' because it is twisted).	If ultrafiltrate could not flow into the PCT, the Bowman's capsule would fill up until no more ultrafiltrate could be formed. Filtration would cease.

As the ultrafiltrate flows past them, cells of the PCT catch solutes and pass them back to the blood. Water follows the solutes by osmosis. This process is REABSORPTION. The PCT usually reabsorbs all the protein and glucose that were in the ultrafiltrate, and it also reabsorbs about 65-80% of Na^+, K^+, Ca^{2+}, Cl^-, HCO3-, and many other ions – and a lot of water. The PCT also moves some compounds from the blood into the ultrafiltrate. This process is called SECRETION. For instance, the PCT secretes aspirin and penicillin into the urine.	If the ultrafiltrate contains too many solutes for the PCT to reabsorb, those solutes will pass out in the urine. For instance, in diabetics the ultrafiltrate may contain more glucose than the PCT can reabsorb. If the PCT cells don't work properly, ions and water won't be reabsorbed as effectively, and will be lost in the urine.
After the PCT, the remaining ultrafiltrate flows down into the LOOP OF HENLE (LOH or nephron loop), which runs down into the center area of the kidney (the RENAL MEDULLA) and up again. The LOH pumps Na^+ and Cl^- out of the ultrafiltrate into the renal medulla. Not much water follows, though, because part of the LOH is waterproof. As a result, the renal medulla becomes salty and hypertonic.	If the LOH doesn't work, the renal medulla will not become hypertonic. This will affect your ability to reabsorb water later on down the nephron.
The ultrafiltrate now flows into the DISTAL CONVOLUTED TUBULE (DCT). The DCT reabsorbs Na^+, Cl^-, and Ca^{2+} (if PTH is present). The end of the DCT, where it attaches to the collecting duct, contains the Na^+/K^+ ATPase that can be activated by ALDOSTERONE. Using this ATPase, the DCT cells can reabsorb Na^+ and water and secrete K^+.	If the Na^+/K^+ ATPase didn't work, you wouldn't be able to reabsorb Na^+ and water when you needed to increase your blood volume. You also wouldn't be able to secrete K^+ when you had too much K^+ in your blood.

Finally, the ultrafiltrate runs down the COLLECTING DUCT to the renal calyx. The collecting duct passes through the hypertonic renal medulla. The Collecting duct is usually pretty waterproof, letting the ultrafiltrate in it run straight out of the kidney. If you secrete ANTIDIURETIC HORMONE, however, the collecting duct becomes permeable to water. Then osmosis will make the water in the ultrafiltrate move out into the hypertonic renal medulla, and it will be reabsorbed into the blood.	If you didn't make enough ADH, your collecting ducts would not be sufficiently permeable to water and you would lose too much water in your urine. You'd become dehydrated. If you made too much ADH, your collecting ducts would be too permeable and you would reabsorb excess water, diluting your blood and making your cells swell. If the renal medulla weren't hypertonic, you would not be able to reabsorb water from the collecting duct effectively and would become dehydrated.
The kidneys help regulate blood pressure by changing the amount of water they filter and reabsorb.	If the kidneys don't produce urine, the blood volume will go up and so will the blood pressure. If they don't reabsorb water, the blood volume and blood pressure will go down.
A special set of cells in the kidneys, the JUXTAGLOMERULAR APPARATUS, measures blood flow in the afferent arterioles and urine Na^+ in the distal convoluted tubule. When blood flow is too high, these cells constrict the afferent arterioles. When blood flow is too low, or the urine flowing past them contains too little Na^+, these cells release renin, which starts the RENIN-ANGIOTENSIN-ALDOSTERONE SYSTEM. One result of this system is to create ALDOSTERONE, which activates the Na^+/K^+ ATPase. Using this ATPase, the DCT cells can reabsorb Na^+ and water and secrete K^+.	Without the juxtaglomerular apparatus, you would not be able to appropriately control the afferent arterioles and adjust the glomerular filtration rate to keep your blood volume normal. You also wouldn't be able to secrete renin and start the RAAS. So your kidneys would stop helping you to maintain your blood pressure. You would keep losing water and Na^+ in your urine, even when you were dehydrated.
The kidneys also control the red blood cell count. When the oxygen levels in the kidneys decrease, they secrete ERYTHROPOIETIN which stimulated RBC production in the bone marrow.	If the kidneys don't produce ERYTHROPOIETIN, your RBC count will decrease and you'll develop anemia. If the kidneys produce too much ERYTHROPOIETIN, your RBC count will increase and it may make your blood too viscous (thick and sticky).
Kidneys activate VITAMIN D3, which is needed for you to absorb Ca^{2+} from your diet.	If the kidneys don't activate Vit D, the calcium you eat will be lost in your stools. Your bones will eventually become weak from not having enough calcium.

Test yourself! Kidney Function and Renal Disorders

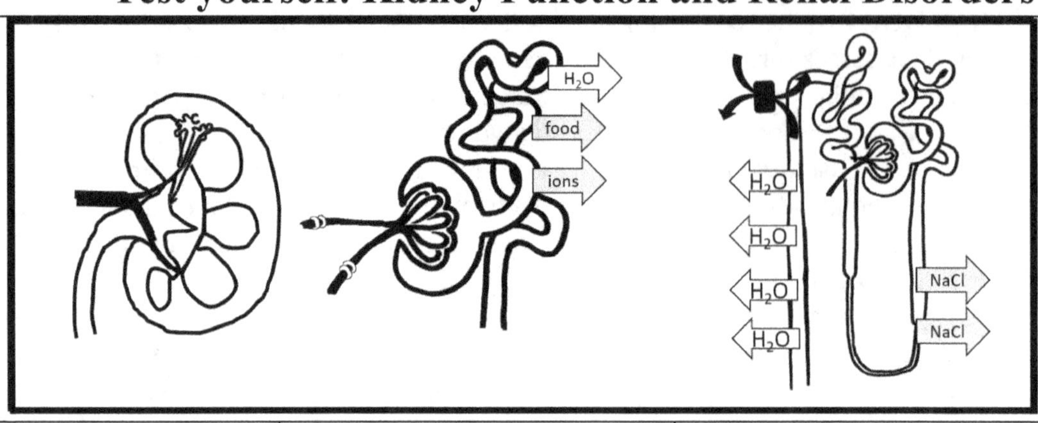

Here's one of your kidneys, filtering your blood. The blood enters through the ________________, which branches until it forms many ________________. Each of these sends blood into a tiny capillary bed called a ________________. After it's been filtered, the blood leaves through the ________________, which return it to the ________________.

The total amount of blood filtered in all these capillary beds is called the ________________ filtration rate, and it is about _____ mL/minute.

The outer layer of the kidneys, containing the filters, is called the ________. The salty inner layer is the ________________.

Here's one of your renal tubules, or ____________. Each of these gets ultrafiltrate from its own ________________. At the other end, the tubule empties urine into the renal ________, which sends it down the ____________ to the ________________. The first part of the tubule, ________________, collects the ultrafiltrate. Everything in the blood except ________, ________________ and ________ can pass through the filter into the ultrafiltrate, but about _____% of the solutes and water are reabsorbed in the ________________. More Na⁺ and water can also be reabsorbed in the ____________, but only if the hormone ________________ has turned on the ________ATPase. This ATPase is also used to remove ______ from the blood.

When ultrafiltrate passes through the Loop of ________, Na⁺ and Cl- are reabsorbed into the renal ____________, making it ________________. This is important because later, when ultrafiltrate passes down the ________________ through this area, water can be ____________ from the urine into the medulla by osmosis. That will only happen if the hormone ________ has made the duct permeable to water. The kidneys respond to low blood flow in the ____________ arteriole by secreting ________, which activates the ________ system and increases ________________ secretion so that the ________ ATPase will reabsorb ____________, making blood volume go _____. If blood O₂ levels are low, the kidneys secrete ________________________ to stimulate RBC production in the bone marrow. And the kidneys activate ____________, which is needed for you to absorb ______ from your diet.

The Bridge Between – Motor Function and Motor Disorders

Normal motor function	What if it goes wrong?
Movement begins with UPPER MOTOR NEURONS in your MOTOR CORTEX. This area is located in the frontal lobe of your CEREBRUM, and has specific cells responsible for movement of different parts of the body.	Without a motor cortex, you'd be unable to move. If you lost the cells responsible for a particular part of the body, you would lose the ability to do voluntary movements of that part of the body.
The motor cortex is on the surface of your brain, so for the impulses to reach your body they must dive down through the brain. Most of them pass along nerve fibers that go through an area called the INTERNAL CAPSULE.	If something damaged the internal capsule, voluntary motor function would be impaired (Puig *et al.,* 2011).
The motor impulses now pass down to the spinal cord. Most of them cross over to the other side of the spinal cord.	This means that damage to the right side of your motor cortex would cause motor impairment on the left side of your body.
As well as the spinal cord, the motor impulses go to the THALAMUS (Bosch-Bouju, Hyland, & Parr-Brownlie, 2013) and some groups of nerve cells called the BASAL GANGLIA. These structures control whether the movement the motor cortex has planned will actually take place. When you're at rest, the basal ganglia release the inhibitory neurotransmitter Gamma-amino-butyric acid, or GABA. This prevents many movements from actually happening. When the basal ganglia release the neurotransmitter DOPAMINE, it tells the thalamus to send messages up to the motor cortex that reinforce the planned movement. Then movement occurs.	Without GABA in the basal ganglia, you would perform random movements all the time. Without Dopamine in the basal ganglia, you would not be able to make the movements you thought of making.
The Cerebellum also contributes to motor impulses at this level, by communicating with the thalamus. It helps with patterned impulses necessary for coordinated motions and learned skills.	Damage to the cerebellum interferes with balance and with the performance of accurate, coordinated movements.

Axons from the motor cortex run down the WHITE MATTER of the spinal cord, carrying the motor impulses. The white matter is called white because of the MYELIN layer that coats each axon, making it possible for nerve impulses to run down the axons very fast.	If the white matter were damaged, you would lose the ability to send motor messages to the body below the area of damage. You would also stop receiving sensory messages from below the lesion. If the myelin were lost, the nerve impulses would not reach the muscles at the right time and movement would become impaired.
When they reach the level of the structure they are sending a message to, these axons synapse with LOWER MOTOR NEURONS in the gray matter of the spinal cord. Lower motor neurons send their axons out of the spinal cord in the SPINAL NERVES. These pass between the vertebrae.	If your vertebrae slipped out of alignment or your intervertebral disks bulged, they could pinch the spinal nerves. Then you would experience pain, numbness, and/or weakness in the part of the body that spinal nerve innervated. If your lower motor neurons were destroyed, you wouldn't be able to send messages to the muscles they control (Knierem, 1997-2017).
Lower motor neurons aren't just responsible for sending the message out to the muscles. They interact with each other to control SPINAL REFLEXES. Some of these reflexes are: The knee-jerk reflex The Babinski reflex The maintenance of muscle tone The patterned gait generator Sympathetic system activation The upper motor neurons can modify these reflexes, but many reflexes will continue without any input from the brain.	If you lost upper motor neuron control of a part of the body but the lower motor neurons remained, so would the spinal reflexes. They might become stronger, because the upper motor neurons would not be inhibiting them. If you lost the lower motor neurons, the spinal reflexes would also be lost (Purves *et al.*, 2001)
Each of the lower motor neurons sends its own axon out in the myelinated spinal nerve, and that axon branches until it synapses with skeletal muscle cells.	If the myelin were lost, the nerve impulses would not reach the muscles at the right time and movement would become impaired.
A lower motor neuron and the muscle cells it controls are called a MOTOR UNIT.	If the motor unit is large, that means a lot of muscles would contract as a unit. For fine movement, you need small motor units so you can move the muscles independently.

At the neuromuscular synapse, the motor neuron releases the neurotransmitter ACETYLCHOLINE, which diffuses over to acetylcholine receptors on the muscle cells. These are called NICOTINIC RECEPTORS.	If you couldn't release acetylcholine, you would not be able to make the muscles contract. If you didn't have acetylcholine receptors, the muscles wouldn't respond to the acetylcholine.
When acetylcholine attaches to the receptors, the muscle cells open their Na^+ channels and Na^+ diffuses in, making the cells depolarize (Greig & Jones, 2016).	If the muscles couldn't open their Na^+ channels, they would not depolarize or contract.
Inside the muscle, Ca^{2+} is released from the sarcoplasmic reticulum and allows the actin and myosin to attach to one another and pull, contracting the muscle.	If too much Ca^{2+} were released, the muscles might contract too much (Greig & Jones, 2016).
The acetylcholine is then removed from the receptors by ACETYLCHOLINESTERASE, allowing the muscle to stop firing and relax.	If there weren't enough acetylcholinesterase, muscles could continue firing for longer (Greig & Jones, 2016).

Bosch-Bouju, C., Hyland, B. I., & Parr-Brownlie, L. C. (2013). Motor thalamus integration of cortical, cerebellar and basal ganglia information: implications for normal and parkinsonian conditions. *Frontiers in Computational Neuroscience*, 7. https://doi.org/10.3389/fncom.2013.00163

Greig, C. A., & Jones, D. A. (2016). Muscle physiology and contraction. Surgery (Oxford), 34(3), 107–114. https://doi.org/10.1016/j.mpsur.2016.01.004

Knierem, J. (1997 - 2017). Disorders of the Motor System (Section 3, Chapter 6) Neuroscience Online: An Electronic Textbook for the Neurosciences | Department of Neurobiology and Anatomy - The University of Texas Medical School at Houston. Retrieved May 1, 2017, from http://neuroscience.uth.tmc.edu/s3/chapter06.html

Puig, J., Pedraza, S., Blasco, G., Daunis-i-Estadella, J., Prados, F., Remollo, S., … Serena, J. (2011). Acute Damage to the Posterior Limb of the Internal Capsule on Diffusion Tensor Tractography as an Early Imaging Predictor of Motor Outcome after Stroke. American Journal of Neuroradiology, 32(5), 857–863. https://doi.org/10.3174/ajnr.A2400

Purves, D., Augustine, G. J., Fitzpatrick, D., Katz, L. C., LaMantia, A.-S., McNamara, J. O., & Williams, S. M. (2001). The Lower Motor Neuron Syndrome. Retrieved from https://www.ncbi.nlm.nih.gov/books/NBK11019/

Test yourself! Motor Function and Motor Disorders

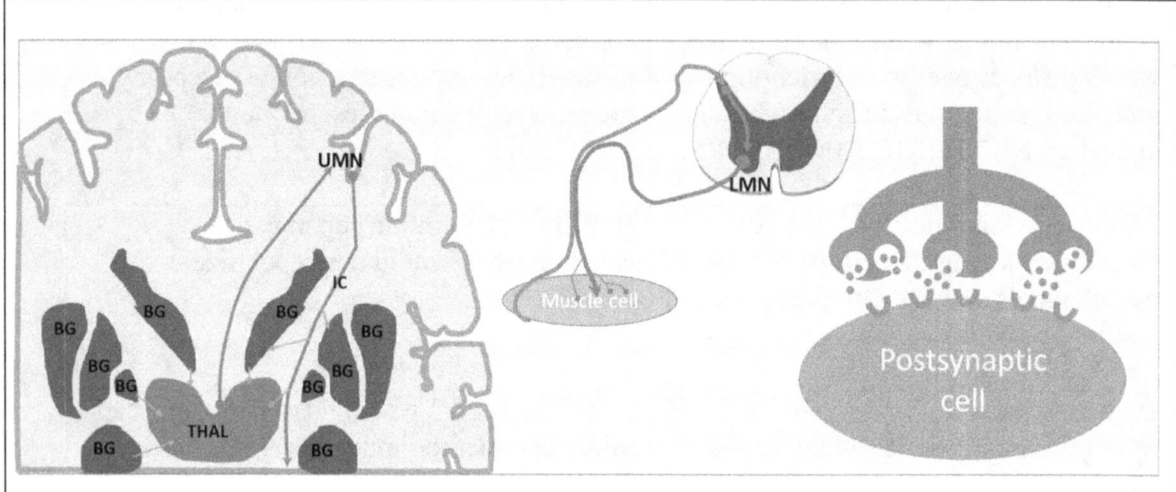

Here are the

____

neurons in your

________________________ . Each
of them controls a specific
part of your body.
To do that, they have to send
their axons down through the
________________________ to the
____________ matter of the
________________________ .

The motor impulses are also
sent to the ____________ and
________________________ ,
which control whether the
movement can occur. The
neurotransmitter __________
prevents unplanned
movements, while the
neurotransmitter

____

reinforces planned
movements.

The axons synapse with

____

neurons living in the

____
of the spinal cord.
These neurons interact
with each other to run
spinal reflexes like the
B________________________
reflex, m____________
t________ , and
p________________________ .
These don't need your
brain to work, but your
upper motor neurons
can modulate them.
Axons from the

____

neurons leave the spine
as the ____________ roots
of the nerves.

Axons from the

____

neurons make up the
____________ nerves,
which carry the signal to
the muscles. To make the
signal move fast enough,
these nerves are coated
with __________ .
The muscle cells controlled
by each neuron are
its________________________ .
They will all contract
together when that neuron
fires.
The neuron makes them
fire by releasing

________________________ ,

which lands on __________
receptors on the muscle
cells and makes them
____________ . The
____________ is then
removed by the enzyme

________________________ ,

and the muscle can relax.

Apply it! Motor Function and Motor Disorders

Mrs. B is 72 years old and complains of leg weakness. She says it's been getting progressively worse. The doctor and the Physician Assistant are discussing her case and they've come up with a list of diseases to investigate and try to rule out.
How could each of these diseases have caused her leg weakness?

Stroke is when a clot or a broken blood vessel cuts off the oxygen supply to cells in the cerebral cortex, killing or injuring them.

Parkinson's Disease is when the basal ganglia lose their ability to make dopamine.

Multiple sclerosis is when axons in the central nervous system begin to lose their myelin coating.

Myasthenia gravis is a disorder that destroys nicotinic receptors on the skeletal muscle cells.

Answer Keys

Key for Stress Response and Stress

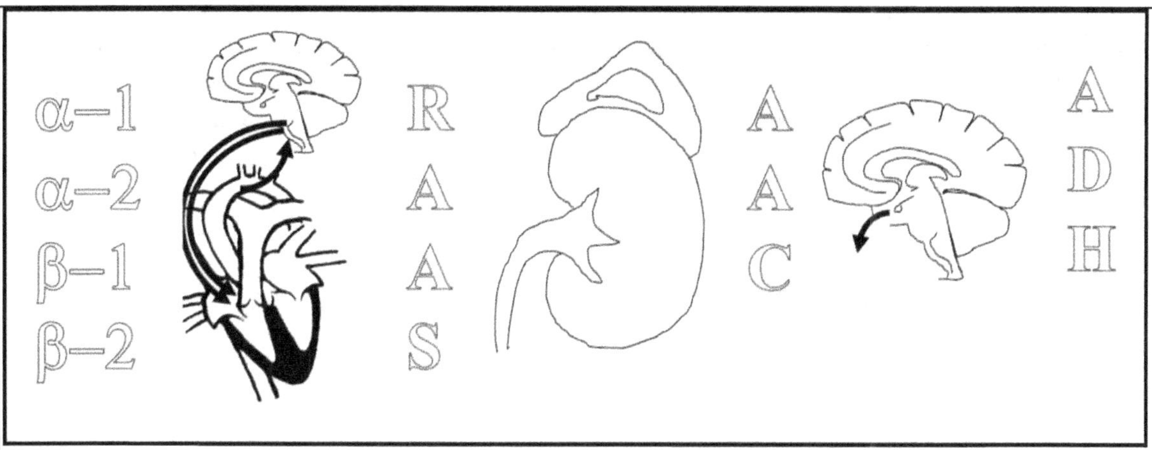

Here's your brain, noticing that you're in trouble.

You might have <u>pain, fear, stress,</u> or <u>low blood pressure</u>. These problems will make the brain turn on the <u>sympathetic</u> nervous system, which will release <u>norepinephrine/noradrenaline</u> from neurons to the target cells and make the adrenal medulla put **EPINEPHRINE/ ADRENALINE** into the blood.

When these compounds attach to <u>alpha-1</u> receptors, blood vessels in the <u>skin, guts,</u> and <u>kidneys</u> constrict. <u>Beta-1</u> receptors make the heartbeat faster and stronger. Beta-2 receptors dilate blood vessels in <u>muscles</u> so you can run away faster, and <u>dilate</u> bronchioles so you can breathe more easily. And <u>alpha-2</u> receptors inhibit further release of <u>norepinephrine</u>, so the system doesn't run out of control.

Your kidneys also notice a problem; their blood flow has <u>decreased</u>!

Special cells called <u>juxtaglomerular</u> cells release <u>renin</u> into the blood. This enzyme converts <u>angiotensinogen</u> into **ANGIOTENSIN I** and the **ANGIOTENSIN** <u>converting</u> enzyme in the lungs further converts that into **ANGIOTENSIN II.**

ANGIOTENSIN II helps raise your blood pressure by making you <u>thirsty</u>, by <u>constricting</u> blood vessels, and by causing the kidneys to <u>reabsorb more</u> Na^+ <u>and water.</u> It also causes **ALDOSTERONE** to be secreted from your adrenal <u>cortex</u>. **ALDOSTERONE** makes the kidneys <u>reabsorb</u> Na^+ <u>and water</u> and <u>secrete K+</u> into the urine.

Your adrenal gland is really busy helping with the stress response.

The adrenal <u>medulla</u> is releasing **EPINEPHRINE** to help the SNS. The adrenal <u>cortex</u> is releasing **ALDOSTERONE** to help the RAAS. And the adrenal cortex is also releasingCORTISOL, the stress hormone that <u>raises</u> your blood glucose and suppresses your <u>immune</u> response.

The last part of the generalized stress response is **ANTIDIURETIC HORMONE**, which is released from the hypothalamus. This causes your kidneys to reabsorb <u>water</u> from your urine into the blood, <u>increasing</u> blood volume.

Mr. O went buffalo hunting, but the buffalo got him instead! His buddies had to drive him back to the nearest town, and he was losing blood all the way. When he arrived at the ER he was pale and his skin was cold; he had a rapid heartbeat and his blood glucose was elevated. Which part(s) of the generalized stress response were causing this? What made them turn on and how were they causing his signs and symptoms?

His sympathetic system has been activated by the fear, pain, and stress of being attacked by a buffalo.CORTISOL release has been activated by stress.

The sympathetic system is releasing norepinephrine and that causes the adrenal medulla to release EPINEPHRINE. Both of these compounds are attaching to receptors in his body.

The alpha-1 receptors are constricting blood vessels in his skin, causing pale and cold skin

The beta-1 receptors are increasing his heart rate.

The alpha-2 receptors are decreasing his INSULIN production, causing his blood glucose to rise.CORTISOL is also raising his blood glucose.

Though it took them two hours to reach the hospital and he drank a whole bottle of water, Mr. O didn't produce any urine on the way. What prevented him from producing urine? What made him thirsty?

Mr. O's sympathetic system will have constricted blood vessels in his kidney, so less blood is reaching kidney tissues. The SNS and the decreased blood supply stimulated his kidneys to secrete renin, which reacted with angiotensinogen to form ANGIOTENSIN I. That then became ANGIOTENSIN II, which caused him to feel thirsty.

The ANGIOTENSIN II caused him to secrete ALDOSTERONE, which made him reabsorb Na^+ from his urine. Water followed it, reducing his urine volume.

He was also secreting ANTIDIURETIC HORMONE (ADH), which caused his kidneys to reabsorb water from his urine into his blood, further reducing urine volume – and keeping him from losing any of the water he drank in his urine.

The medical team sprang into action, stopping his bleeding and giving him an IV to replace blood volume. An hour later, he was more comfortable – but he still hadn't produced any urine. The med student said "That's normal, isn't it?" "Just barely," said the doctor. "I'm getting worried about it."
What could happen to Mr. O if his stress response stays on for too long?

The biggest risk is probably to his kidneys, which have had their blood flow reduced for a while now! They could suffer from decreased oxygen. His GI tract is facing the same challenge, since the SNS vasoconstricted it. If the SNS kept stimulating his heart, it could become damaged as well; the harder it works the more oxygen it will need!

Key for Inflammation and Inflammatory Disorders

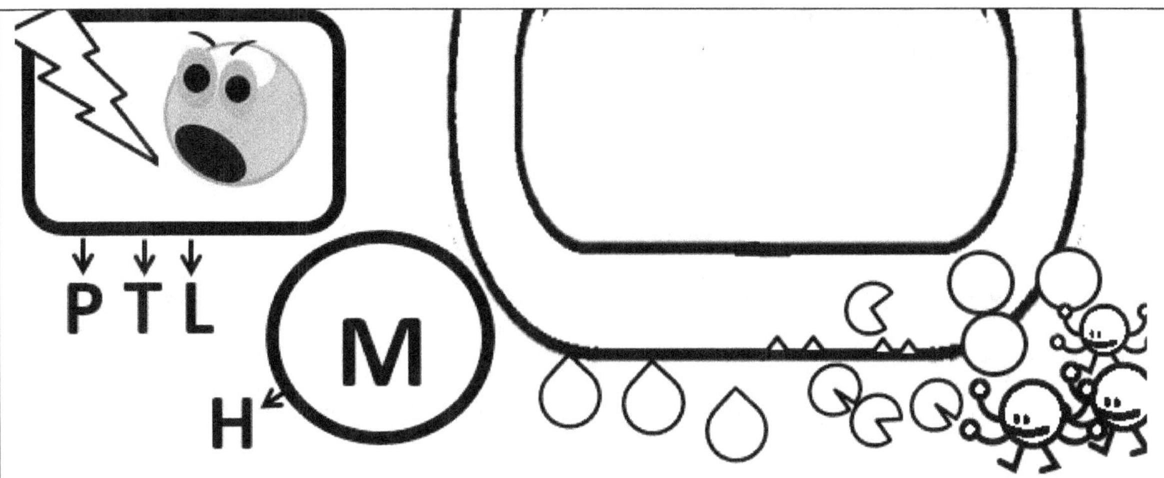

Here's your poor sad cell, damaged by some awful trauma!
The cell will turn <u>arachidonic</u> acid from its membrane into inflammatory mediators. These include <u>prostaglandins</u>, <u>leukotrienes</u>, and <u>thromboxane A2</u> .

White blood cells (WBCs) called <u>mast cells</u> are also living in the tissue, and they respond to the injury by releasing more inflammatory mediators, including <u>histamine</u>.
One of these inflammatory mediators, <u>thromboxane A2</u>, will increase clotting in the injured area.

Here comes a blood vessel running through your injured tissue. All those inflammatory mediators will make it <u>vasodilate</u>, bringing in more blood.
It will also become more <u>permeable</u> , letting fluids leak out into the tissues.
This response is called the <u>vascular response</u>, and it can, if widespread, <u>decrease</u> blood volume and blood pressure.

On its inside lining, the blood vessel will begin to produce <u>adhesive</u> proteins to catch passing WBCs.

The first WBCs to enter the injured area are the <u>neutrophils</u>. They eat pathogens and secrete many chemicals, including <u>enzymes</u> that can break down damaged tissue.

The second wave of WBCs to reach the area includes <u>monocytes</u>, which mature into <u>macrophages</u> when they enter the tissue.
They will secrete many compounds, including <u>cytokines</u> which cause a fever, <u>increased</u> WBC count, and other signs of an <u>acute-phase</u> or <u>systemic inflammatory</u> response.

Key for Immune System and Immune Disorders

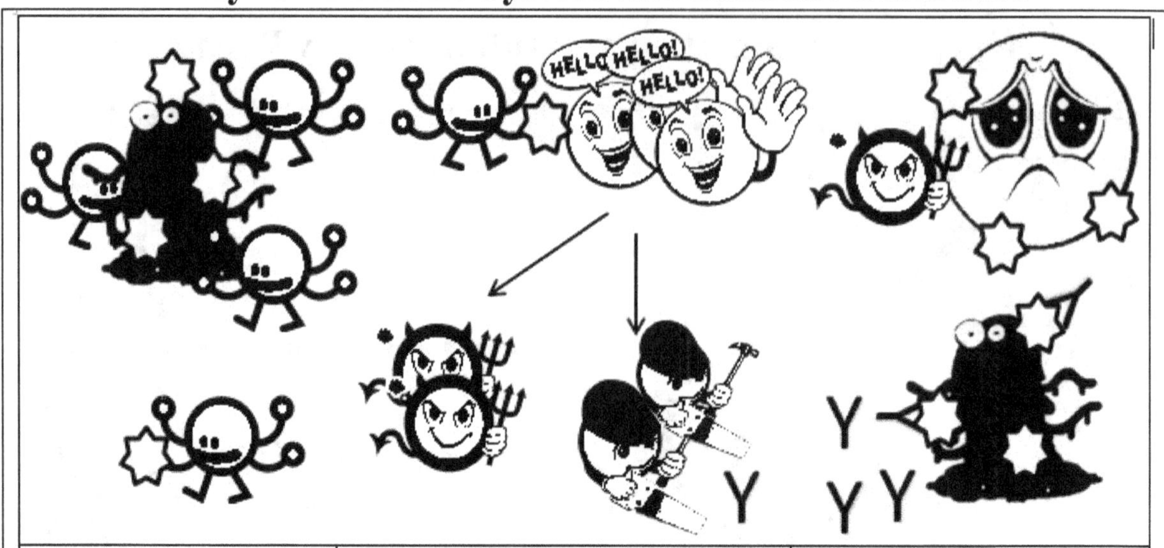

Here's a horrible virus attacking your tissues! You can identify it by the <u>antigens</u> on its surface.
It begins an inflammation, which attracts <u>antigen-presenting cells</u>.
They eat the pathogen and display the <u>antigens</u> on their <u>MHC II</u> proteins.

Now these <u>APCs</u> will enter a lymph vessel and travel up to the <u>lymph node</u>, where they will present the <u>antigen</u> to the immune cells, or <u>lymphocytes</u>.

Here we are in the lymph node, and the <u>T helper</u> cells (also called CD4$^+$) are looking at the <u>antigen</u>. If one of them has a receptor that matches it, that cell will begin to divide and secrete <u>cytokines</u>. It will stimulate the <u>T cytotoxic</u> cells and the <u>B</u> cells that have the same receptor, and start them dividing too.

The <u>T cytotoxic</u> cells, also known as CD8$^+$, will go out into the blood searching for cells making the <u>antigen</u>. They will look for it on the <u>MHC I</u> proteins on the surfaces of your cells.

The <u>B</u> cells will create special proteins that can attach to the <u>antigen</u>. These proteins are called <u>antibodies</u> or <u>immunoglobulins</u>.

Here's a poor sick cell infected with a virus. See the viral <u>antigen</u> on its
<u>MHC I</u> proteins? When the <u>T cytotoxic</u> cell detects that, it will kill this infected cell.

Meanwhile, any antigens outside the cell are being attacked by the <u>antibodies</u>. They will mark the virus to be eaten by <u>white blood cells</u> or destroyed by the protein <u>complement</u>.
Soon you're well! And if you meet this infection again, you have <u>antibodies</u> and <u>memory cells</u> just waiting to destroy it.

Images from Microsoft Clip Art, 2013

Mrs. V retired to her dream home in the country, but she ran into trouble as soon as spring came and the trees bloomed. "All it took was one whiff of pollen, and my nose turned into a fountain!" she says. "Antihistamines are my new drug of choice."
What is making her nose run, and how do antihistamines relieve it?

Her runny nose is due to the vascular response of inflammation. Mast cells in her nasal tissues are releasing inflammatory mediators. These mediators include prostaglandins, leukotrienes, and histamine. They make her blood vessels dilate, bringing lots of blood to her nose, and make her capillaries permeable so fluid and protein can leak out of those blood vessels. That exudate is dripping out of her nose, and the antihistamines will help stop the vessel dilation and permeability that's causing it.
But antihistamines will not address the underlying allergy that makes this happen.

Blood tests showed that Mrs. V had anti-birch pollen antibodies in her blood. She doesn't understand how these got there. How did she develop these antibodies, and how did they begin an inflammation?

At some time, Mrs. V was exposed to birch pollen and some of it got into her blood, where it was recognized as foreign and eaten by an antigen-presenting cell. The APC carried the pollen's surface antigens up to a lymph node, where a browsing T helper cell with a receptor that fit onto the antigen stimulated an immune response. The Th cell divided into other T cells, including Th2 cells, which stimulated B cells to divide into plasma cells and create antibody proteins that fit onto the birch pollen antigen. Some of these antibodies attached to Mast cells, making them respond to the pollen and cause an inflammation.*

The birch trees stopped blooming, and Mrs. V got out in the back yard. There, she discovered a new problem – poison ivy! Her back yard was full of it, and even though she wore gloves and was very careful while she cleared it out, she got a rash. She complained to her doctor about this allergy that was making her sick over and over. "This isn't the same allergy," the doctor said. "For one thing, the antigen you're reacting against is different. For another, this rash is caused by T cytotoxic cells, not by antibodies."
What are T cytotoxic cells, how did she get them, and how are they causing a rash?

At some time, Mrs. V was exposed to poison ivy and some of its compounds got into her blood, where they were recognized as foreign and eaten by an antigen-presenting cell. The APC carried the poison ivy antigens up to a lymph node, where a browsing T helper cell with a receptor that fit onto the antigen stimulated an immune response. The Th cell divided into other T cells, including Th1 cells. These stimulated T cytotoxic cells to go out in the body and search for body cells 'infected' with the poison ivy antigen. Those Tc cells are attacking any of her own skin cells that have the poison ivy antigen on them.
**By the way, in cases of allergy like these, where the body is over-reacting to something that's not really dangerous, the antigen is called an 'allergen.'*

Key for Hemostasis and Clotting Disorders

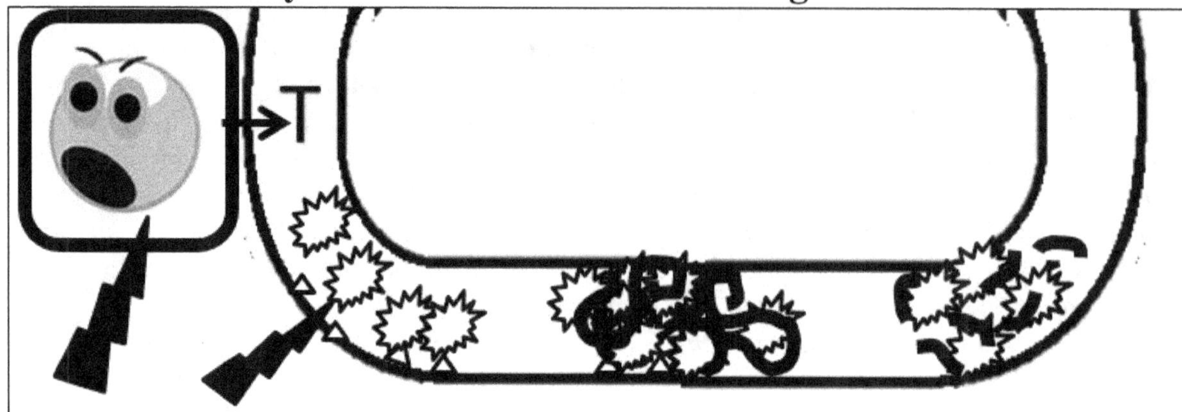

Here's your poor sad cell, damaged by some awful trauma!
The cell will create inflammatory mediators. These include <u>thromboxane A2</u>, which increases platelet function.

Your blood vessel has been damaged too. Some of its cells are broken, and the collagen underneath is showing through.

Platelets, or <u>thrombocytes</u>, attach to the damaged area. They need <u>von Willebrand</u> factor to attach to collagen.

Compounds from the injured blood vessel (the <u>intrinsic</u> system) and from damaged tissues (the <u>extrinsic</u> system) activate <u>procoagulation</u> factors in the bloodstream. Many of these are proteins that were synthesized by the <u>liver</u>. Vitamin <u>K</u> is needed to synthesize them, and <u>calcium</u> is needed for them to work.

The <u>procoagulation</u> factors activate the enzyme <u>thrombin</u>, which turns <u>fibrinogen</u> in the blood into <u>fibrin</u> filaments.
These filaments then tie the platelets together into a strong clot.

Clot production is kept from going too far by <u>anticoagulation</u> factors made in the liver.

The clot breaks down when tissue <u>plasminogen</u> activator turns the blood protein <u>plasminogen</u> into the enzyme <u>plasmin</u>, which breaks the <u>fibrin</u> strands apart.

Sad cell from Microsoft clip art, 2013

Mr. G is in the hospital because of complications associated with liver and kidney failure. His blood results are way off; he has high levels of waste products in his blood, very low platelet and erythrocyte counts, and low calcium.
The doctors are discussing whether he should be put on dialysis to clean the wastes out of his blood.
Doctor Bob says, "I'm worried about his bleeding too much." Why is Dr. Bob worried about bleeding?
The liver produces many compounds needed for clotting: thrombopoietin, which causes platelet formation, and many procoagulation factors. The kidneys are the other main source of THROMBOPOETIN, but Mr. G's kidneys are also failing.
Without thrombopoietin, Mr. G has developed a low platelet count and that will decrease his ability to clot. He is also probably not producing enough procoagulation factors to promote clotting.
In addition, his calcium is low. Calcium is needed for proper function of some of the procoagulation factors.

Doctor Sue says, "There's recent work suggesting that liver failure can cause too much clotting, though." How could liver failure increase clotting?
The liver produces anticoagulation factors as well as procoagulation factors. With a failing liver, Mr. G might make too few anticoagulation factors, so he might clot too much.

"That's true," says Dr. Bob, "but his med history shows that he's also been taking a lot of aspirin." Why is this relevant?
Aspirin attaches to platelets and prevents them from making thromboxane A2, so they are unable to stick together and form clots. The few platelets Mr. G has may be useless for clot formation, if they have aspirin attached to them.
Doctors have to take a lot of factors into consideration when deciding how to deal with potentially altered clotting in patients with liver failure, because with the liver producing fewer pro- and anticoagulation factors, the patient loses much of their ability to appropriately regulate clot formation (Lisman and Porte, 2017).

Lisman, T., & Porte, R. J. (2017). Pathogenesis, prevention, and management of bleeding and thrombosis in patients with liver diseases. *Research and Practice in Thrombosis and Haemostasis*, *1*(2), 150–161. https://doi.org/10.1002/rth2.12028

Key for Red Blood Cells and Anemias

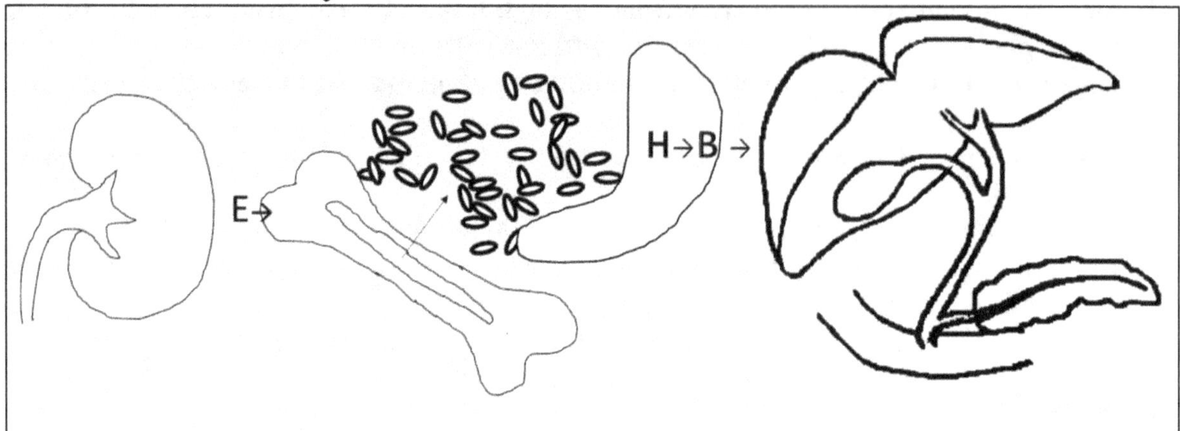

Here's your poor sad kidney, not getting as much oxygen as it wants. It's going to secrete the hormone **ERYTHROPOIETIN**, which will travel through the blood to your <u>red bone marrow</u> and stimulate it to create <u>RBCs</u> .	Here's your bone. The bone <u>marrow</u> is busy creating more RBCs. When the RBCs are still immature they have <u>organelles or nuclei</u>, but as they mature they lose these, until the almost-mature RBCs (called <u>reticulocytes)</u> only have their <u>endoplasmic reticulum</u>. Then that is lost also and the mature RBC (called an <u>erythrocyte)</u> is filled with <u>hemoglobin</u>.	Here are your mature RBCs (called <u>erythrocytes</u>) floating in the blood. When they are worn out they'll be destroyed by the <u>spleen</u> and the heme portion of the hemoglobin inside them will be turned into <u>bilirubin</u>. The liver will use this to make <u>bile</u> and store it in your <u>gall bladder</u>.

Mr. A has an inherited condition that damages the membranes on his RBCs, causing them to develop an abnormal shape and wear out too quickly. Why has he developed anemia?
Mr. A's red blood cells are wearing out too quickly, faster than he can replace them.
Therefore he is running out of RBCs in his circulation.
This is hemolytic anemia, which means the problem is that the cells are breaking too much.

The doctor is checking Mr. A's liver and spleen. Why does the doctor expect them to be enlarged?
Since the spleen breaks RBCs, it will be overworked and become enlarged in a disease where too many RBCs are being broken.
The liver has to deal with all the bilirubin being produced as the spleen breaks down all those RBCs – so the liver also is enlarged.

Now the doctor has ordered blood tests for erythrocytes, reticulocytes, and ERYTHROPOIETIN. What do you expect the results to be like? Why?
The mature RBC (erythrocyte) levels will be low, because they are being destroyed.
There will be more immature RBCs (reticulocytes) than usual – because the bone marrow is trying to replace the destroyed erythrocytes as fast as it can, releasing lots of reticulocytes.
Since there are fewer RBCs than usual, there is probably less oxygen reaching the kidneys – and they will be secreting ERYTHROPOIETIN. So that level will be higher than normal.

Key for Osmosis and Fluid Imbalance

Here's the water you drank, in your GI tract. It can only get into your blood by <u>osmosis</u> . That's easy if all you did was drink, because drinking water made your GI contents <u>hypo</u>tonic to your blood, and water will move <u>into</u> the blood.

If you ate food as well, your GI contents contains solutes (S) and may be <u>hyper</u>tonic to your blood. Then water will move from the <u>blood</u> into the <u>GI contents</u>.

As your small intestine absorbs the food into the blood, water will <u>follow</u> the food solutes back into the blood.

In the large intestine, you'll absorb <u>ions</u> from the GI contents into the blood. Water will <u>follow</u> those solutes too, ending up in the <u>blood</u>.

Here's a blood vessel flowing through your tissue. As your blood passes through tissues, <u>blood pressure</u> pushes some of the water out of the vessel into the <u>intercellular</u> space.

If too much water enters the <u>intercellular</u> space, that tissue could develop <u>edema or swelling</u>.

But water is removed by the <u>lymph</u> vessel at the bottom of the picture, which sends it to the <u>lymph nodes</u> and then back into the venous blood. Finally, water from your blood filters into the urine in your kidneys.

If your body is dehydrated, cells in your hypothalamus will <u>shrink</u>. This stimulates the hypothalamus to start the <u>thirst</u> response and to secrete <u>ADH</u>, a hormone which makes your kidneys reabsorb water into your blood.
The water added to your blood will make the blood <u>hypotonic</u> and the hypothalamus cells will <u>swell</u>, shutting off the response.

Water can also be reabsorbed from the kidneys by the <u>RAA</u> system, which activates Na^+/K^+ ATPase. This protein moves
<u>2 K⁺</u> from the blood into the urine and <u>3 Na⁺</u> from the urine into the blood. Water follows the <u>3 Na⁺</u> back into the blood, increasing blood <u>volume</u>.

Mr. D has diabetes insipidus – he can't make ADH. How will this affect his ability to control blood osmolarity?
Without ADH, he can't reabsorb water from his urine into his blood. So water will be lost in his urine, and his blood will contain less water. It will be hyperosmolar.

One of the side effects of diabetes insipidus is constant thirst. How is the disorder leading to this effect?
Thirst happens when the blood becomes hyperosmolar to cells in the hypothalamus, causing water to move out of those cells and make them shrink. Since he's unable to keep water in his blood, Mr. D's blood is likely to be hyperosmolar and his hypothalamus cells are constantly shrinking.

Another side effect of diabetes insipidus is constant urination. Mr. D has this too! How was it caused?
Since he's unable to reabsorb water from his urine into the blood, the water stays in his urine. That means his urine volume will be high, and the urine will be very dilute.

Mr. D has been coping with his disease very well, just by adjusting his behavior. But then he caught the 'stomach flu' and spent two days sick in bed. He says he was barely able to get to the toilet fast enough to throw up. He ran a high fever and his respiration rate increased, as well. Then he had cold sweats. Right now he says he feels horrible, and when you check his vitals you see that his eyes are sunken, his lips are dry, his pulse is rapid and weak and his blood pressure is dangerously low. What has happened to his water balance, and why?
Mr. D's been losing water lots of ways. First, through vomiting. Then the high fever and increased respiration rate caused him to lose more water by evaporation from his lungs. The sweating made him lose water by evaporation from his skin. And because he was throwing up, he wasn't able to use the behavioral adjustment – drinking – that kept him hydrated before he got ill. As a result, his blood volume is dangerously low and his cells are shrinking, causing his sunken eyes and dry lips.

Mr. D's wife had the same 'stomach flu,' but although she threw up just as much and had the same fever, her blood pressure is almost normal. Why?
Mrs. D was throwing up and losing water from her lungs and skin, but because her brain could secrete ADH she was able to recover some water from her urine. This means her situation isn't as bad.

Key for Potassium and Potassium Imbalance

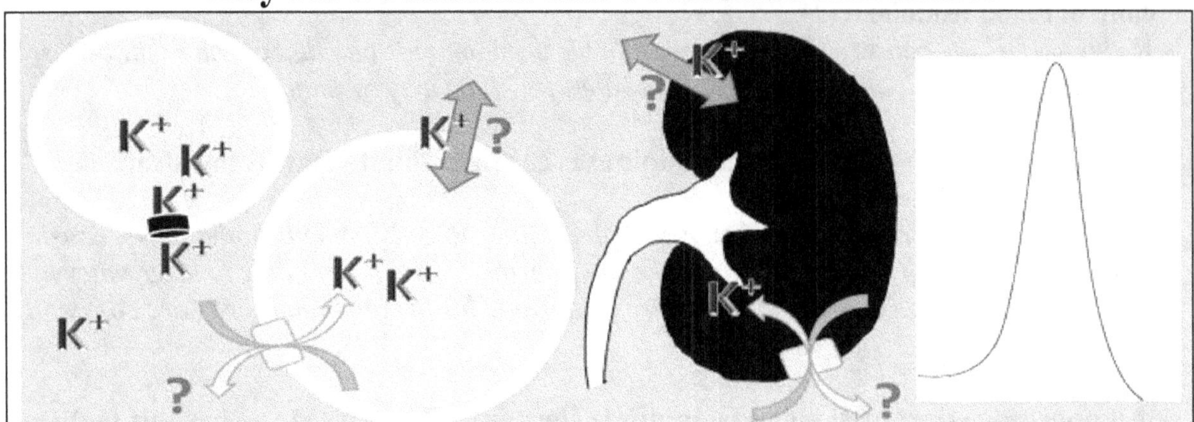

Here's the K^+ you ate, absorbed into your blood. But most of the K^+ will move into your <u>cells</u>. It can move back out of your cells by diffusing through special proteins called <u>K^+ channels</u>. Because this movement is driven by the concentration difference between K+ inside and outside your cells, blood K^+ levels can affect your cell K^+ levels. If blood K^+ increases, intracellular K^+ will <u>increase</u>.	Your cells can pick up K^+ actively, as well. They do this with the Na^+/K^+ ATPase protein, which moves <u>2 K^+</u> into the cell and <u>3 Na^+</u> out of the cell. This ATPase is activated by <u>INSULIN</u> and the <u>SNS</u>. Your cells can also pick up K^+ with the $K^+/\underline{H^+}$ exchange. This pump is reversible! It can pick up K^+ from the blood, or release it into the blood. When you use it, though, you will change your blood's <u>pH</u> levels.	You get rid of excess K^+ through your kidneys. They also have a <u>Na^+/K^+</u> ATPase protein. This protein moves <u>2 K^+</u> from the blood into the urine and <u>3 Na^+</u> from the urine into the blood. The <u>K^+</u> is then lost in the urine. The renal $\underline{Na^+/K^+}$ ATPase is activated by the hormone <u>ALDOSTERONE</u>. Kidneys also have a reversible $K^+/\underline{H^+}$ exchange.	The biggest effect K^+ has on your cells is by raising or lowering their <u>resting potential</u> Too much K^+ in the blood makes cells <u>hypopolarized</u>, bringing their charge nearer to <u>threshold</u>. They'll fire <u>too easily</u>. Too little K^+ in the blood will <u>hyper</u>polarize your cells, bringing their charge further away from <u>threshold</u>. Their firing will <u>decrease</u>.

Mr. K has diabetes mellitus – he can't make INSULIN. How will this affect his ability to move K^+ from his blood into his cells?
Insulin normally activates the Na^+/K^+ ATPase, which moves K^+ from the blood into the cells. Without INSULIN, Mr. K isn't able to activate that pump as much as usual – so more of the K^+ is staying out in his blood. He is at risk for hyperkalemia, or high potassium in the blood.

One of the side effects of diabetes mellitus is ketoacidosis, a condition in which there is too much H^+ in the blood. Mr. K has developed this condition. How will his cells correct it, and what will happen to his blood K^+ levels as a result?
Your cells use the H^+/K^+ exchange to regulate blood K^+ levels, but they also use it to regulate blood H^+ levels.
Mr. K has too much H^+ in his blood, so the cells will pick some of it up using their H^+/K^+ exchanges. When they pick up the H^+, though, that means they must release K^+ into the blood. Mr. K's blood K^+ levels will go up!

Another side effect of diabetes mellitus is kidney failure. Mr. K has this too! How will it affect his blood K^+ levels?
The kidneys are really good at cleaning K^+ out of your blood. But if Mr. K's kidneys aren't working, they can't do this job properly – K^+ will build up in his blood because he can't get rid of it through his urine.

Mr. K is feeling very strange. Sometimes his heart feels like it's missing beats, and sometimes his legs cramp up. The doctor ordered an EKG and when it came back, she was really concerned. She said his heart wasn't firing normally. How could his K^+ levels be involved in this?
Mr. K's blood K^+ levels are going up and up – and so is the resting potential of his nerve and muscle cells. They will fire too quickly, and respond to every little stimulus. Mr. K's leg muscles are contracting too much, and his heartbeat is irregular. If his K^+ goes much higher, he'll go into cardiac arrest! (This is why K^+ is used for lethal injections.)

The doctor treated Mr. K with INSULIN. The med student wanted to know if they shouldn't give him some ALDOSTERONE to fix his K^+ levels, but the doctor said INSULIN would be enough. Would ALDOSTERONE have been a good idea?
ALDOSTERONE makes your kidneys run their Na^+/K^+ ATPase, which will move K^+ from the blood to the urine. It would have been a good idea, but Mr. K's kidneys aren't working! So the INSULIN, which will make his cells pick up K^+ from his blood, is a better idea.

Key for Calcium and Calcium Imbalance

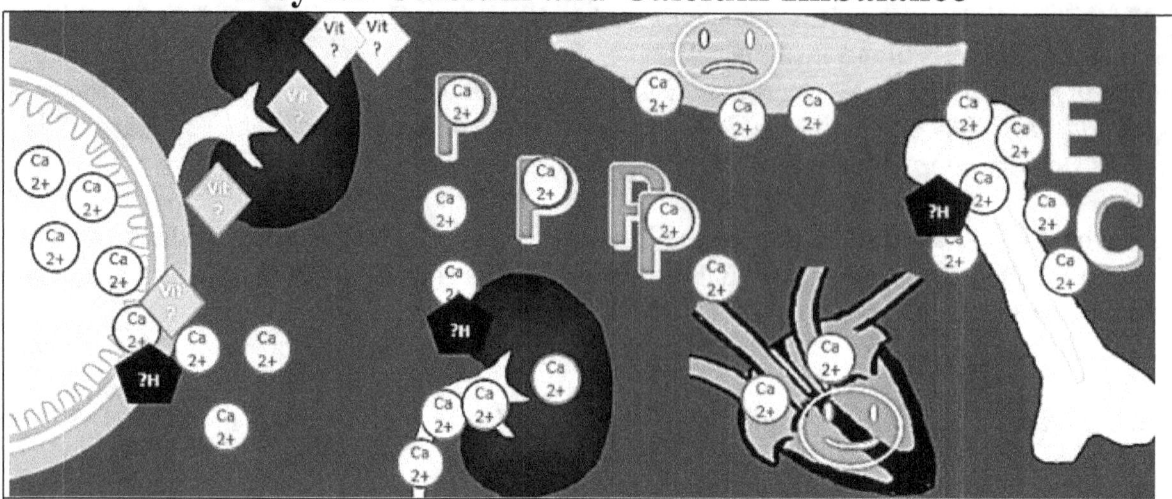

Here's your intestine, full of the dairy products you ate.
If you have enough **PARATHYROID HORMONE** and activated vitamin **D3**, you can absorb the calcium from this food into your blood.

You can get that vitamin **D3** from your diet if you are able to digest **fats**. Or you can make it in your **skin**, if there's enough **sunlight**. Either way, the vitamin **D3** must be activated by your **kidneys** before it will help you absorb calcium from your diet into your blood.

Here are the calcium ions absorbed into your blood. About half of them will bind to **protein** The other half become the Ca^{2+} ion, and are called **ionized** calcium. Some of the calcium filters out of the blood into your kidneys, and is lost in your **urine.**

When the calcium ions attach to the outside of skeletal muscle cells, they block the Na^+ channels and make it harder for the muscle to fire.

But the heart and **smooth** muscles have special proteins called **calcium channels,** which let the calcium into the cell. Once inside these cells, calcium will make them contract **more strongly.**

The hormones **ESTROGEN** and **THYROCALCITONIN** help your bones store calcium. Load-bearing **exercise** does it too!

When blood calcium is low, your **parathyroids** secrete **PTH**. At first, this hormone stimulates the bone-building cells. If it remains elevated, though, it has a different effect. If **PTH** remains elevated, it will help you absorb Ca^{2+} from your intestines, reabsorb it from your urine, and release it from your bones into the blood.

Mr. P has kidney failure. How will this affect his ability to absorb calcium from his diet?
His kidneys can't activate enough vitamin D3 → he can't absorb enough calcium from his diet

The medical student expected Mr. P to develop low blood calcium, so she did a neurological test to check. If he has low blood calcium, will he develop stronger or weaker reflexes? Why?
Normal: *calcium in the blood attaches to the outside of nerve and skeletal muscle cells → blocks the Na^+ channels → making it hard for the cells to fire*
If Mr. P doesn't have enough calcium in the blood → fewer Na^+ channels will be blocked → nerves and muscles will fire more easily → reflexes will be stronger

The medical student was surprised to find Mr. P's reflexes normal. She ordered an analysis of his blood and found that his blood calcium levels were normal! Where could he be getting the calcium to keep his blood levels normal?
When blood calcium levels are decreasing, he can release calcium from his bones into the blood. Or he could reabsorb it from his urine into the blood.

The medical student ordered measurements of Mr. P's PARATHYROID HORMONE levels. Do you think they are high or low? Why?
Normal: *When blood calcium decreases → Parathyroid glands release PTH → which causes bones to release calcium into the blood, increases calcium absorption in the GI tract, and makes you reabsorb more calcium from the urine.*
Mr. P can't absorb enough calcium from his diet, so his calcium levels probably started to go down. That caused his parathyroids to secrete PTH. You would expect him to have elevated PTH right now, because he is using this system to keep his blood calcium normal.

Before the test results came back, Mr. P stubbed his toe while going to the bathroom. His foot is really sore and his toe is swollen. The medical student says this injury isn't related to his calcium balance, since his reflexes were normal. The nurse thinks it might be related. How might it be related?
The student is thinking about why Mr. P might have had motor problems. It's true that his blood calcium is probably not making him stumble and run into things, since his calcium levels and his reflexes are both normal.
But the nurse is thinking about his bones. He's releasing calcium from his bones into his blood. This will make his bones weaker, so that stubbed toe might actually be a broken toe!

Key for Acid, Base, and Acid-Base Imbalances

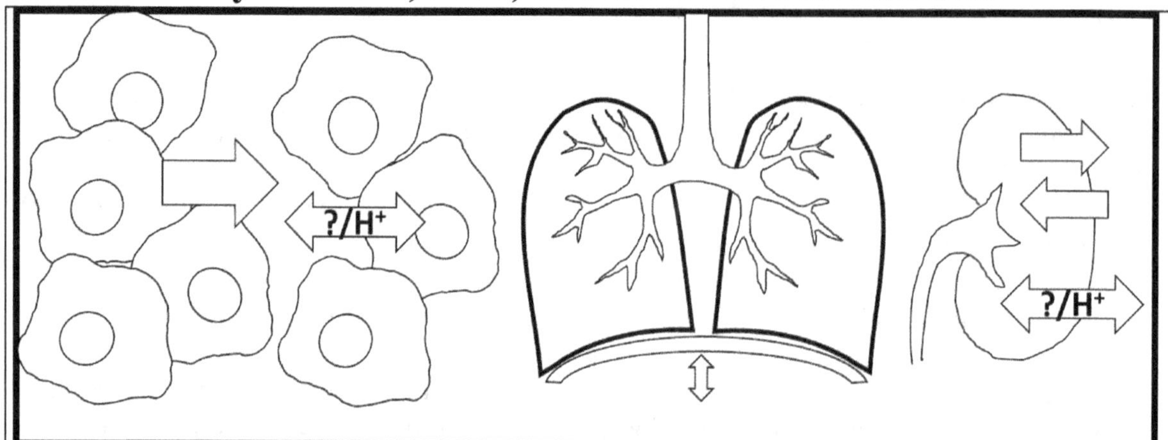

Here are your busy cells, producing all kinds of acids!

They're producing a lot of CO_2, the volatile acid. They're also producing nonvolatile acids like lactic acid, ketoacids, and hydrochloric acid.

CO_2 actually becomes an acid when it combines with H2O in the bloodstream to become carbonic acid.

All these acids can affect your blood pH because they release H^+ ions.

They didn't make your blood pH change too much, though, because most of those H^+ ions combined with buffer molecules in your blood. The major molecules performing this function are proteins and bicarbonate.

Here are your cells again, trying to regulate the acid levels in the blood.

They can do this by picking up or releasing H^+ ions – but they must exchange them for K^+ ions.

If your cells pick up H^+ from your blood, they will release K^+ into your blood.

When the blood reaches your lungs, the carbonic acid breaks apart again into CO_2 and H2O. These are removed from the blood when you exhale.

To make sure you do this enough, you regulate your breathing based on blood CO_2 and pH. You will breathe more if CO_2 is high or pH is low.

Here's your kidney, filtering the acids and bicarbonate out of your blood.

The kidneys can raise your blood pH by sending the H^+ ions into the urine, but putting the bicarbonate back into the blood.

Kidneys can also adjust blood H^+ by exchanging it for K^+, just like your cells.

With so many ways to adjust blood pH, you manage to keep it stable. That's important because H^+ ions will decrease nerve and muscle firing, if they build up in your blood.

Mrs. T had a panic attack, which made her breathe way too fast. What happened to her blood pH? Which acid was affected, and how?
The rapid breathing allowed Mrs. T's lungs to exhale more CO_2 than usual. As a result, she removed the volatile acid from her blood and her blood became more basic – the pH increased.

Mrs. T began to suffer some side effects from her altered blood pH. How did the panic attack change the concentration of H^+ in her blood, and what did that do to her nerves and muscles?
The concentration of H^+ in Mrs T's blood was too low, because she was exhaling too much volatile acid. H^+ in the blood decreases nerve and muscle firing, so when the H^+ levels in the blood decreased, Mrs. T's nerves and muscles were able to fire more than usual. Her reflexes probably got stronger, and she could have developed spasms from the muscle firing, and tingling from the nerve firing.

When her blood pH began to change, Mrs. T's cells responded to adjust it. How did that change her blood K^+ levels?
Mrs. T's cells detected the high pH outside and began to release H^+ from inside the cells into the blood. This brought the pH back down. But when they released H^+, the cells had to exchange it for K^+. They picked up K^+ from the blood, and her blood K^+ levels decreased.

Mrs. T's kidneys also adjusted her blood pH. What were three ways they could do this?
Mrs. T's kidneys were filtering her blood, removing both H^+ and buffers like bicarbonate. They responded to her high blood pH by returning some of the H^+ to the blood, and letting the bicarbonate go out in the urine.
Also, her kidneys did the same thing her cells were doing – they exchanged H^+ for K^+, putting more H^+ back into the blood and moving K^+ from the blood into the urine.

Key for Breathing and Respiratory Disorders

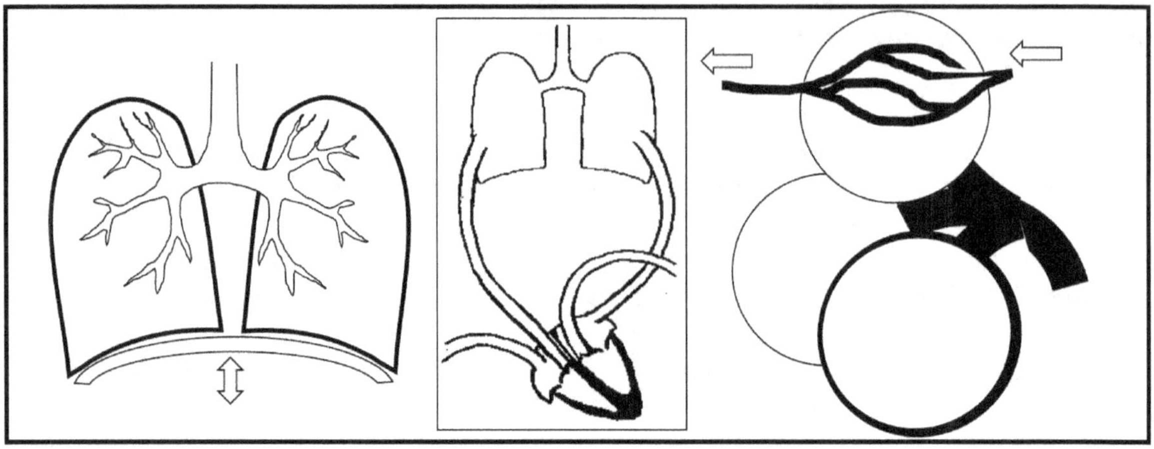

Here are your lungs, attached to your airway. When you move air into and out of the lungs, it is called <u>ventilation</u>.

To move air into your lungs you contract your <u>diaphragm</u> to lower the floor of your chest cavity, making more room for air. You can also expand the walls of the chest cavity using your <u>accessory</u> muscles.

You need to inhale enough air to fill your <u>dead space</u> and then your <u>respiratory zone</u>. The soapy substance inside the alveoli, <u>surfactant,</u> allows your lungs to expand easily as you inhale.

The <u>right</u> side of your heart pumps blood to your lungs through the <u>pulmonary</u> trunk and arteries.
After the arteries come the <u>pulmonary</u> <u>arterioles</u> and the <u>pulmonary</u> <u>capillaries</u>.

Perfusion of the lungs is controlled by vasodilation and vasoconstriction. In areas of the lung where there is a lot of O_2 and not very much CO_2, vessels <u>dilate</u>. In areas where there is not much O_2 but a lot of CO_2, vessels <u>constrict</u>.
This process is called <u>ventilation-perfusion</u> <u>matching</u>, and ensures that more blood goes to the areas with fresh air.

Your respiration rate is controlled by two sets of <u>chemoreceptors</u>. The <u>central</u> sensors respond to <u>low pH</u> levels in your <u>cerebrospinal fluid</u>. When you accumulate CO_2 in your blood, some of it is converted into <u>carbonic acid</u> and causes the pH to <u>decrease</u>. These sensors will then cause respiration to <u>increase</u>, exhaling more CO_2 and making the pH <u>go back up</u>.

The <u>peripheral</u> sensors are located in your <u>aorta</u> and <u>carotid arteries</u>. They stimulate breathing when blood O_2 levels <u>decrease</u>.

Mr. S is a fireman who was caught in a collapsing building. He arrived at the emergency room unconscious, with three broken ribs and a sucking chest wound. The EMT had put a dressing over the chest wound. She says, "I don't think we got it fast enough; the lung on this side is collapsed."
A sucking chest wound is an injury that lets air move through a hole in the chest wall into the pleural space outside the lungs. Why would this make the lung collapse?
As air came in through the hole in the chest wall, it accumulated in the pleural space OUTSIDE the lung. The air filled up the space, and left no room for the lung to expand. Doctors will be able to fix this pretty simply, by putting a tube in to drain the bubble of air out of the chest.

Doctors inserted a chest tube to remove the air in Mr. S's chest cavity, and his lung reinflated. But later that night, he began to complain of respiratory distress. His pulse oximeter showed a steady decrease, and his lungs sounded wet. "That's what I was afraid of," said one of the nurses. "He inhaled smoke, and now he might be developing ARDS."
In Acute Respiratory Distress Syndrome (ARDS), one problem is that the surfactant in much of the lung tissue is destroyed. Why is this dangerous?
Surfactant is the soapy substance that lines your alveoli, reducing the attraction of water molecules to one another so that your alveoli are able to expand when you inhale. Mr. S has lost the surfactant in many of his alveoli, so the water molecules inside those alveoli are sticking together so strongly that he isn't able to expand the alveoli. The effect has been to reduce the working portion of his lungs. He's trying to get oxygen with smaller working lungs, so of course he is having a hard time.

The doctor has Mr. S transferred to the ICU. "We need to measure his pulmonary blood pressure, because it might spike," the doctor says. Why might Mr. S's pulmonary blood pressure go up?
Pulmonary blood vessels dilate in parts of the lung that contain O_2, and constrict in parts of the lung that don't contain much O_2. That normally works well, sending the blood to the places where it will pick up O_2. But in Mr. S, much of his lungs no longer contains O_2 – so most of his pulmonary vessels will constrict, pushing his pulmonary blood pressure up. Increased pulmonary blood pressure is found in most cases of ARDS (Ryan, Frohlich, and McLoughlin, 2014).

Ryan, D., Frohlich, S., & McLoughlin, P. (2014). Pulmonary vascular dysfunction in ARDS. *Annals of Intensive Care, 4*, 28. https://doi.org/10.1186/s13613-014-0028-6

Key for Heart Function and Cardiac Disorders

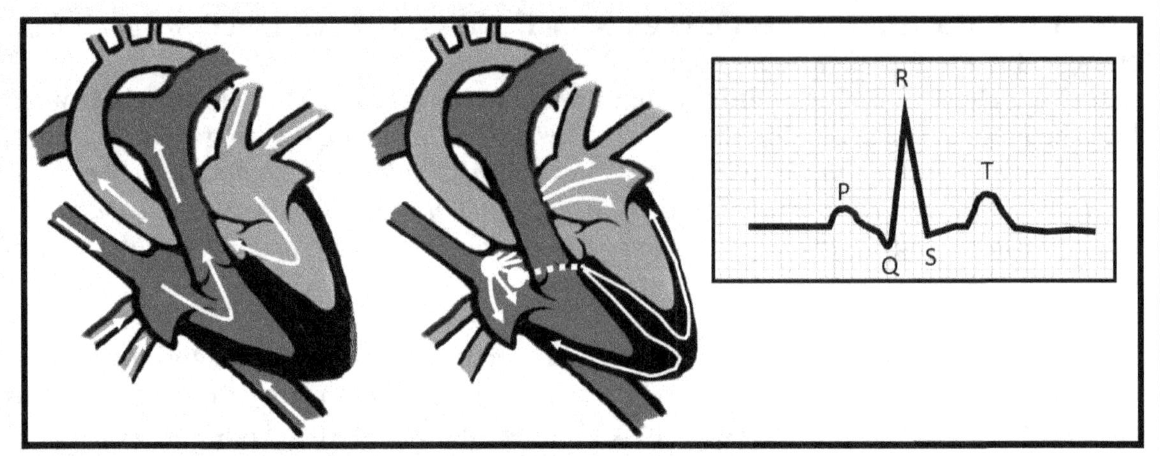

Here's your heart, divided into the right and left sides. Blood from the body enters the <u>right atrium</u>, passes through the <u>tricuspid</u> valve, and goes into the <u>right ventricle</u>. When the heart contracts during <u>systole</u>, that blood will be pushed out into the <u>pulmonary</u> circuit.

At the same time, blood from the lungs is entering the <u>left atrium</u> and going down through the <u>bicuspid or mitral</u> valve into the <u>left ventricle</u>, which will send it into the <u>systemic</u> circuit.

When the ventricles contract during <u>systole</u>, they push blood up against the <u>bicuspid</u> and <u>tricuspid</u> valves, closing them and causing the first heart sound.

The blood is pushed out of the left ventricle through the <u>aortic semilunar</u> valve and pushed out of the right ventricle through the <u>pulmonary semilunar</u> valve. When the ventricles stop contracting, these valves snap shut, making the second heart sound.

Contraction starts when the <u>SA</u> node depolarizes. It depolarizes automatically, but can be speeded up by the <u>sympathetic</u> system or slowed down by the <u>parasympathetic</u> system.
The impulse spreads across the <u>atria</u>, making them depolarize and causing the <u>P</u> wave of the EKG.

Then the impulse passes through the <u>AV</u> node and Bundle of <u>His</u> into the ventricles. While this is happening, the EKG shows the <u>PR segment</u>.

In the ventricles, the impulse flows along the <u>bundle</u> branches and <u>Purkinje</u> fibers to make the ventricles depolarize.
When ventricles depolarize, you see the <u>QRS complex</u> on the EKG.
Finally, ventricles repolarize again. That causes the <u>T wave</u> on the EKG.

Ms. P has been feeling weak and tired. She also complains of shortness of breath, and sometimes she wakes up at night with a feeling that she's drowning. Her blood pressure is low, her heart rate is high, and her lungs sound wet. Her pulseox is lower than normal, and you hear a murmur between her first and second heart sounds. The doctor orders a bedside ultrasound, and it reveals that Ms. P's aortic valve isn't opening all the way. Her left ventricle is enlarged.

Has the partly blocked aortic valve affected the heart's preload or afterload?
Afterload. The aortic valve doesn't have anything to do with blood entering the heart; it is affecting the amount of work the heart must do to pump that blood out again.

Why is the left ventricle enlarged?
The afterload on the left ventricle has increased, and like any muscle the ventricle muscle becomes larger when it has to work harder. In addition, the left ventricle may be unable to pump out a normal amount of blood through the narrowed aortic valve, so it may be stretching because it contains too much blood.

Why is her blood pressure decreased?
Blood pressure is affected by how much blood the left ventricle can push out into the arteries. With the aortic valve partly blocked, that amount has decreased – and so has the blood pressure.

Why is her heart rate increased?
The decreased blood pressure turned on her sympathetic system, which released norepinephrine to the pacemaker cells in her SA node. The norepinephrine attached to beta-1 receptors, making the pacemaker fire more quickly and increase her heart rate.

The murmur you heard is the sound of turbulent blood forcing its way through the narrowed valve. Do you hear this sound during diastole or during systole? Why? Why do you hear the sound before the second heart sound?
The murmur comes when blood is being forced through the aortic valve. That happens during systole, when the ventricles contract. The sound comes before the second heart sound, because the second heart sound is when the semilunar valves (aortic and pulmonary) close completely – and then you won't hear blood being forced through them any more.

Does the valve defect explain Ms. P's drowning sensation, or is that a separate problem?
The valve defect explains her lung problems. The left heart's job is to take blood from the lungs and pump it out to the body, and the valve defect is preventing the left heart from moving as much blood as it should. As a result, blood accumulates in the lungs. She feels as if she's drowning because she is, in a sense – her lungs are filling with fluid.

Key for Blood Pressure and its Disorders

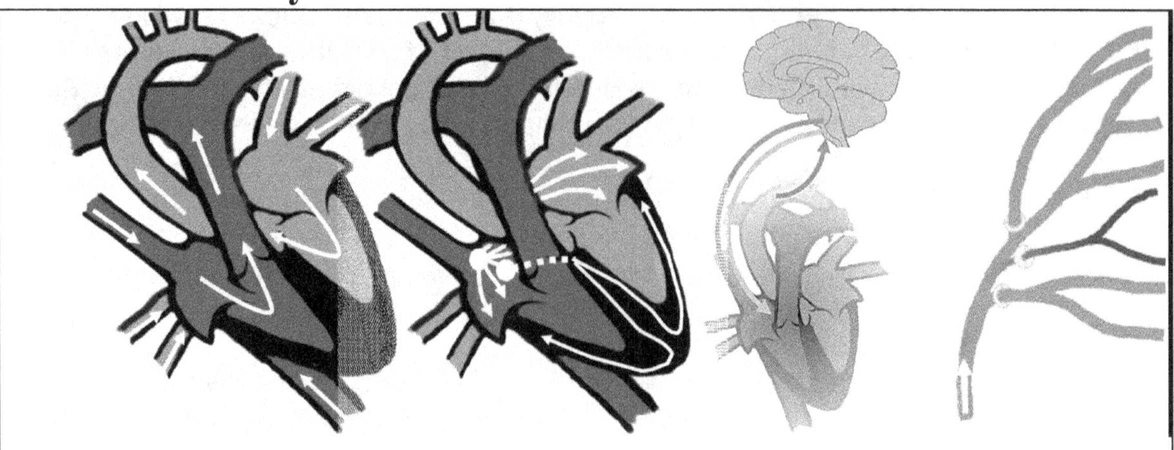

Here's your heart, pumping blood into an artery. The blood presses against the artery walls; this is called the <u>blood pressure</u>.
The amount of blood the heart pumps into the arteries every minute is the <u>cardiac output</u>. It depends on the <u>heart rate</u> and the <u>stroke volume</u>. If the amount of blood pumped goes down, blood pressure will <u>go down</u>. In the artery, the pressure of blood against the artery walls is measured by stretch receptors called <u>baroreceptors</u>. They're located in the <u>carotid</u> arteries and the AORTA.
These receptors send information about the blood pressure to the <u>cardiac control</u> and <u>vasomotor</u> centers in the medulla oblongata.

Here's your medulla, getting messages about the blood pressure and comparing it to the <u>set point</u>.
If BP is too low, the <u>cardiac control</u> center in the medulla will tell the heart to <u>speed up</u>, using neurons from the <u>sympathetic</u> system. If blood pressure is too high, the medulla will tell the heart to <u>slow down</u>, using the <u>parasympathetic</u> system.

The heart isn't the only thing that controls blood pressure. If the blood vessels <u>constrict</u> and get smaller, they will squeeze on the blood and blood pressure will increase. This is called <u>peripheral resistance</u>.

Here's an arteriole with a sphincter around it. The sphincter can open or close to let blood flow into the capillary bed.
If the sphincter opens, the vessel has <u>vasodilated</u>. This will make blood pressure <u>decrease</u>. If the sphincter closes, the vessel has <u>vasoconstricted</u> and the blood pressure will <u>increase</u>.

These sphincters can be controlled by the <u>vasomotor</u> center in the medulla oblongata.
If BP is too low, the <u>vasomotor</u> center will turn up the <u>sympathetic</u> system to make the sphincters <u>vasoconstrict</u>. If BP is too high, it will turn this system down to let the sphincters <u>vasodilate</u>.

A woman having a widespread allergic reaction suffered rapid vasodilation of all her arterioles at once. How will this affect her blood pressure, her medulla oblongata, and her heart rate?

Vasodilation → blood vessels relax → less pressure on blood → low peripheral resistance → low blood pressure.

Baroreceptors report the blood pressure to the medulla oblongata, which compares the blood pressure to the set point and identifies that it is too low. The cardiac control center of the medulla sends impulses down sympathetic nerves to the heart and makes the heart speed up.

The woman injected herself with an epi pen containing EPINEPHRINE, a sympathetic system stimulant. How would this help her?

Epinephrine helps the sympathetic system work harder. Her heart will speed up more, raising cardiac output. Epinephrine will also make sphincters in her arterioles constrict, raising peripheral resistance. Both of these will increase her blood pressure..

When she arrived at the hospital, the doctor noted that her heart rate was very high but her blood pressure was still low. What do you think the woman's peripheral resistance was?

Blood pressure depends on cardiac output and peripheral resistance. Her cardiac output has probably increased, since her heart rate is high. So the only reason for her blood pressure to remain low must be that her peripheral resistance is still low.

After receiving intravenous fluids, the woman's blood pressure increased. Was this because her cardiac output increased, or her peripheral resistance? Why?

Giving fluids increased her blood volume, which increased her stroke volume. Her heart was pumping more blood with every beat, increasing her cardiac output.

The woman's blood pressure got a little too high as she began to recover. What will her medulla oblongata do to bring it down again?

Baroreceptors report the blood pressure to the medulla oblongata, which compares the blood pressure to the set point and identifies that it is too high. The cardiac control center of the medulla sends impulses down parasympathetic nerves to the heart and makes the heart slow down, decreasing cardiac output. The vasomotor center of the medulla decreases sympathetic stimulation of sphincters in the arterioles and makes them vasodilate, lowering peripheral resistance.

With both cardiac output and peripheral resistance decreasing, the blood pressure will decrease.

Key for GI function and GI problems

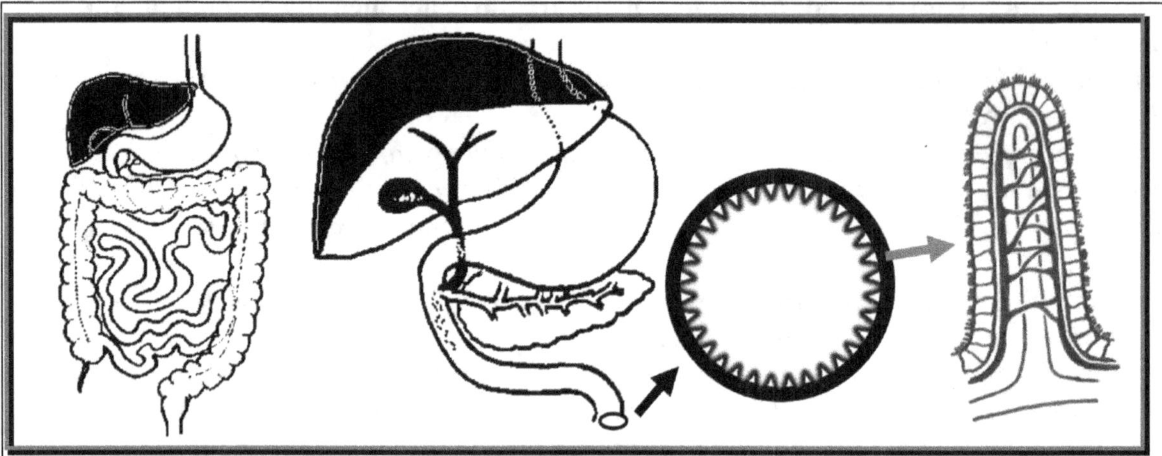

Here's your GI tract, ready to carry out its four functions: <u>motility, secretion, digestion, and absorption.</u>

Swallowing moves food into the <u>esophagus</u>. The food passes through the <u>upper esophageal</u> sphincter into the stomach, where it is mixed with HCl and <u>pepsinogen</u>.
In your stomach, the HCl converts the <u>pepsinogen</u> into <u>pepsin</u>, which begins the digestion of <u>proteins</u>. HCl is also needed for absorption of <u>iron</u>.
The stomach is protected from the HCl by a layer of <u>mucus</u>.
Vit B12 is absorbed using <u>intrinsic factor</u>, which is also produced by the stomach.
As long as food is in the stomach, stomach cells will release the hormone <u>GASTRIN</u>, which stimulates more stomach secretion.

Here's the beginning of your small intestine, where the food will go next.

When food finally leaves the stomach, it will go through the <u>pyloric sphincter</u> into the <u>duodenum</u>. Three digestive hormones are released: <u>GIP</u> causes the body to make INSULIN, <u>SECRETIN</u> turns off stomach secretion and makes the <u>pancreas</u> release bicarbonate (antacid), and <u>CHOLECYSTOKININ</u> makes the gall bladder release <u>bile</u> and the <u>pancreas</u> release digestive enzymes.

Here's a section of your small intestine showing the finger-like <u>villi</u>. Their job is to <u>absorb</u> the food from the intestinal contents and pass it to the blood or lymph.
Food you haven't digested will move through the <u>ileocecal</u> valve into the <u>colon</u>, where bacteria break some of it down and produce <u>gas</u>. This region of the intestine also absorbs <u>water</u> and <u>electrolytes</u> into the blood.
Undigested food passes into the <u>rectum</u> and out the <u>anus</u>.

Key for Liver Function and Liver Failure

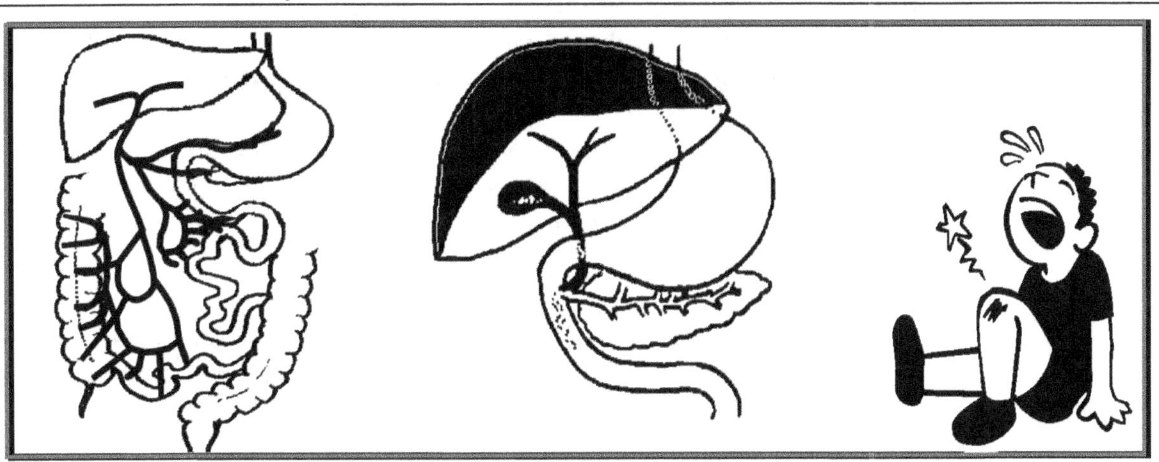

Here's your liver, getting blood from the GI organs through the <u>hepatic portal vein</u>

If you just ate a lot of sugar, the liver will store it as <u>glycogen</u>. But if you haven't eaten, the liver will break the <u>glycogen</u> down and release glucose into your blood.

If you only ate fats and proteins, the liver will convert some of them into <u>glucose</u> to keep your blood levels stable.

It will also make some of the fats and proteins into <u>ketones</u>.

TOXINS! The liver will break these down into <u>water</u>-soluble forms that can be excreted in your urine.

The liver removes bilirubin from the blood and makes it into <u>bile</u>, which is stored in the gall bladder and sent to the intestines where it helps <u>emulsify</u> fats.

The liver converts ammonia into <u>urea</u>

The liver also breaks down hormones like <u>ALDOSTERONE</u>. Without the liver, the Na^+/K^+ ATPase pump in the kidneys would keep running.

Your liver also produces <u>procoagulation</u> and <u>anticoagulation</u> factors. Without these you might bleed too much. – or too little.

Another blood protein the liver produces is <u>albumin</u>, which maintains the blood osmolarity.

The liver packages fats into <u>lipoproteins</u>, which carry them to the cells.

Mr. X has been drinking for years, and his doctor tells him he has alcoholic liver disease and fat malabsorption. Mr. X says this is nonsense, because his problem is booze – not fat! He shows you how thin his arms and legs are. "Not an ounce of fat on 'em!" he says. "That's not what I mean," the doctor says. "I mean you're not digesting the fat you eat." Why can't Mr. X digest fat properly?
Because Mr. X's liver is damaged by dealing with all the alcohol he drinks, it can't keep up with its other jobs. One of those is to make bile, which is needed to emulsify fats in the intestines (break them into little droplets that can be easily digested). The fats aren't being digested, and are going out in Mr. X's stools.

Mr. X has yellow skin and the whites of his eyes are yellow as well. What caused this?
He is jaundiced because his liver isn't able to remove bilirubin from the blood fast enough. The bilirubin is depositing in his skin.

When you look at Mr. X's arms you notice a lot of bruises and some scabs. He says "I have thin skin, I bruise myself all the time." How could his liver disease be related to this?
The liver should be making clotting proteins. Without them, Mr. X bleeds too much whenever he bumps himself. The bleeding under his skin is what's causing all those dark bruises.

The doctor has ordered some blood tests on Mr. X – Potassium (K^+), ammonia, and blood osmolarity. What do you think they will show?
Potassium is a really important test, because an imbalance of K^+ could cause cardiac arrest. Mr. X's liver may not be breaking down ALDOSTERONE, which would mean the ALDOSTERONE stayed in his body and the Na^+/K^+ pump in his kidneys kept running. This pump moves Na^+ into the blood and puts K^+ out in the urine, lowering blood K^+ levels.

The liver should be converting ammonia into urea. If the liver isn't doing its job, the ammonia will build up and eventually be toxic to Mr. X's nerves and brain.

Blood osmolarity controls the movement of water between cells and blood. The blood osmolarity is controlled by the solutes in the blood, and albumin made by the liver is an important one of those solutes. Without enough albumin, the blood will become hypoosmolar – too watery – and water from the blood will start to enter the cells. Mr. X's cells could begin to swell up, and if his brain swells up it could kill him.

Key for Pancreas Function and Pancreatic Disorders

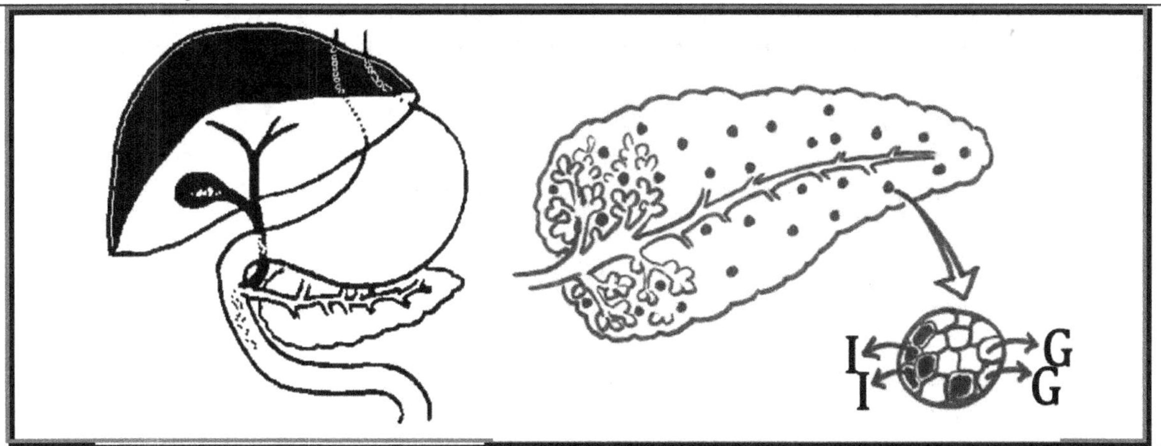

Here's your pancreas, right below your stomach. The <u>exocrine</u> pancreas sends <u>enzymes</u> and <u>bicarbonate</u> through the duct to your duodenum, where they help digest food and <u>neutralize</u> acid.

The <u>endocrine</u> pancreas is not attached to the pancreatic duct. It is made up of the <u>islets of Langerhans</u>, which secrete hormones into the blood.

When you have high blood sugar levels, the <u>beta</u> cells secrete <u>INSULIN</u>, which allows your cells to <u>pick up</u> the sugar from your blood and store it as <u>glycogen</u>.

When your blood glucose levels are low, the <u>alpha</u> cells secrete <u>GLUCAGON</u>, which makes your cells break down food and release it into the blood.

When you're hungry, your cells break stored <u>glycogen</u> into glucose and release it.
They break stored fats into <u>free fatty acids</u> and proteins into <u>amino acids</u>. Your liver will convert some of these into <u>ketoacids</u>.

Blood pH will <u>decrease</u> because of all the <u>acids</u>.

A child has diabetes mellitus and cannot make INSULIN, but he can make GLUCAGON. He comes into hospital with weight loss, high blood glucose, high levels of amino acids and free fatty acids in his blood, high levels of ketones, heavy breathing, and dehydrated cells.

How did his lack of INSULIN contribute to his high blood glucose?

Without INSULIN, his cells are not able to pick up glucose from the blood. The glucose remains in the blood, building up to high levels – sometimes 5-6x normal values!

How did his GLUCAGON contribute to his high blood glucose?

GLUCAGON is a hormone released by the pancreatic alpha cells when they are not getting enough glucose. Because this boy isn't making INSULIN, his pancreatic alpha cells aren't able to pick up glucose, so they begin to release GLUCAGON.

GLUCAGON makes cells that contain stored sugar release it into the blood. It also makes the liver create glucose from other compounds like fatty acids. Therefore, it will contribute to the high glucose in this child (Fanelli et al., 2006).

Which of the two hormones is responsible for his high amino acid, free fatty acid, and ketoacid levels? How?

GLUCAGON is the main hormone involved in this. It makes the cells release stored foods into the blood. Fat is released as free fatty acids, and protein is released as amino acids. GLUCAGON also stimulates the liver to turn the free fatty acids and amino acids into ketoacids.

Which of the two hormones is most responsible for his weight loss? How?

GLUCAGON would be to blame here too, since it makes cells break down and release the foods inside them.

Why are his cells becoming dehydrated? How do you think he will try to compensate for that?

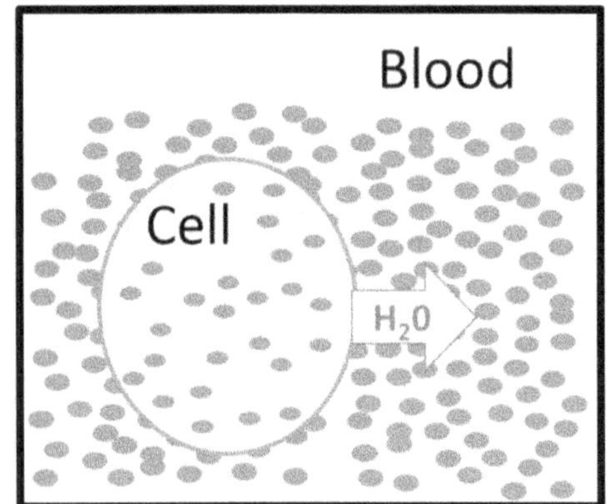

This is an osmosis problem. The glucose, amino acids, free fatty acids, and ketoacids in the blood are all solutes, making the blood hypertonic to the cells. Water leaves the cells by osmosis.

As cells in his hypothalamus shrink, the boy will become thirsty and drink water in an attempt to rehydrate himself.

Fanelli, C. G., Porcellati, F., Rossetti, P., & Bolli, G. B. (2006). Glucagon: the effects of its excess and deficiency on INSULIN action. Nutrition, Metabolism, and Cardiovascular Diseases: NMCD, 16 Suppl 1, S28-34. https://doi.org/10.1016/j.numecd.2005.10.018

Key for Thyroid Function and Thyroid Disorders

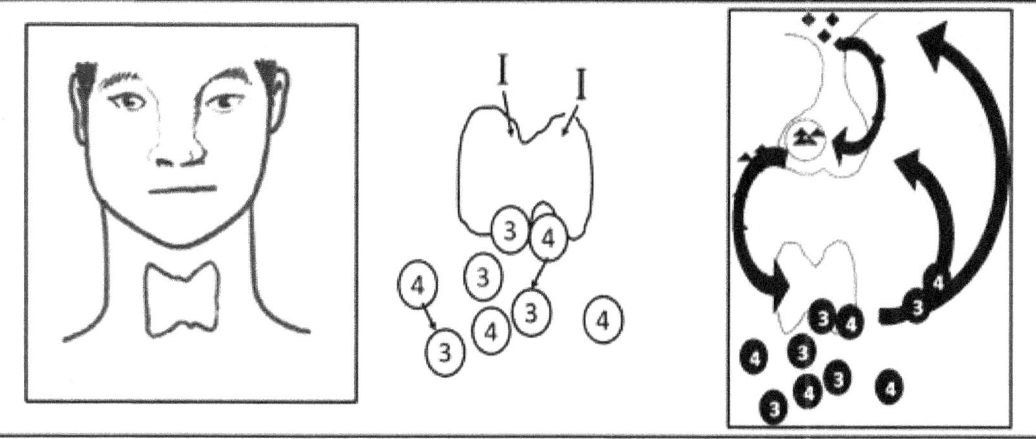

Here's your thyroid, right below your adam's apple. The thyroid releases <u>triiodothyronine</u> and <u>tetra-iodothyronine</u> into your blood.
The active hormone is <u>triiodothyronine</u>, and it <u>increases</u> your metabolic rate by stimulating <u>aerobic</u> respiration. You make <u>more</u> ATP, leading to increased <u>muscle</u> and <u>nerve</u> firing and weight <u>loss</u>.
The other hormone, <u>tetraiodothyronine</u>, is converted into <u>triiodothyronine</u> when your tissues need it.

Your thyroid is controlled by the <u>hypothalamus</u>, a region of your brain that secretes <u>thyrotropin</u> Releasing Hormone when it is stimulated by cold or <u>low</u> levels of <u>triiodothyronine</u> and <u>tetraiodothyronine</u>.
The <u>thyrotropin</u> Releasing Hormone goes to your <u>anterior pituitary</u>, which then releases <u>thyrotropin</u>, or <u>thyroid</u> Stimulating Hormone.

The <u>thyroid</u> Stimulating Hormone travels through the blood to the <u>thyroid</u>, stimulating it to release <u>triiodothyronine</u> and <u>tetraiodothyronine</u>.

The hypothalamus and <u>anterior pituitary</u> continue secreting their Releasing and Stimulating hormones until they detect normal levels of <u>triiodothyronine</u> and <u>tetraiodothyronine</u> in the blood.

Key for Adrenal Cortex Function and Adrenal Disorders

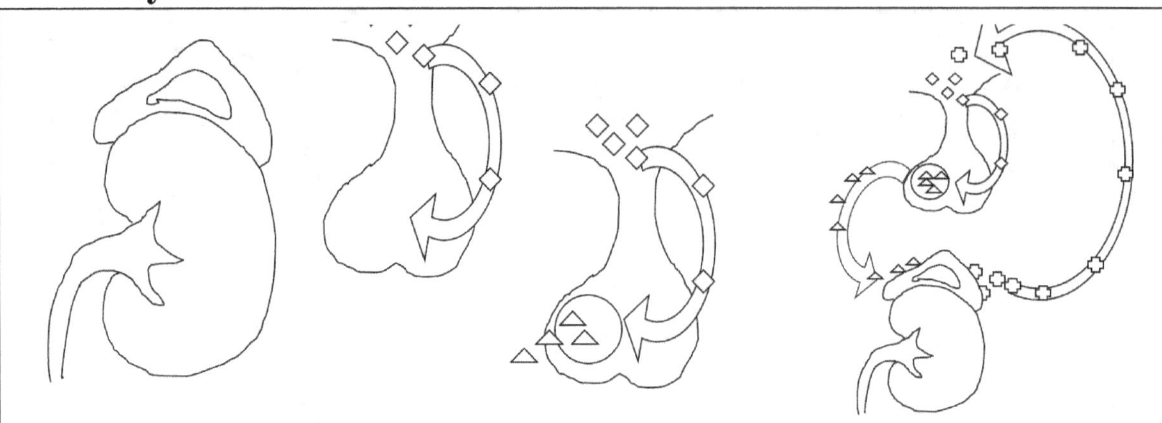

Here are your adrenals, right on top of your kidneys.
The adrenal cortex is the <u>outer</u> layer of each adrenal gland, and it producesCORTISOL, <u>**TESTOSTERONE**</u>, and <u>**ALDOSTERONE**</u>.

When kidneys activate the <u>**RAAS**</u> or blood K^+ levels <u>increase</u>, the adrenal cortex releases <u>**ALDOSTERONE**</u>. This hormone activates the <u>Na^+/K^+ ATPase</u> in the kidneys, causing <u>Na^+</u> to move from the urine to the blood and <u>K^+</u> to move from the blood into the urine.

Adrenal secretion ofCORTISOL is controlled by the <u>hypothalamus</u>, a region of your brain that secretes <u>corticotrophin</u> Releasing Hormone when it is stimulated by stress or <u>low</u> levels ofCORTISOL.

The <u>**corticotrophin**</u> Releasing Hormone goes to your <u>anterior pituitary</u>, which then releases <u>adrenal corticotrophic</u> Hormone.

The ADRENAL CORTICOTROPHIC HORMONE travels through the blood to the <u>adrenal cortex</u>, stimulating it to releaseCORTISOL.

The hypothalamus and <u>**anterior pituitary**</u> continue secreting their Releasing and Stimulating hormones until they detect normal levels ofCORTISOL in the blood.

Cortisol's major effects on a healthy body are to increase its responsiveness to the sympathetic system, to raise blood glucose

A child's parents have brought him in to the clinic because they are afraid he has diabetes mellitus. "He's always urinating, and that's a sign," says his mom. "And he's thirsty all the time."
The doctor asks whether the boy is hungry or losing weight. "He isn't losing weight, but we can't keep him away from the chips and sweets," says his mom. "If we won't let him have snacks, he eats salt right out of the salt shaker!"
The doctor takes the boy's vital signs and observes that his blood pressure is low, and his heart rate is elevated. A blood glucose test shows that the boy's blood glucose is low. "I don't think it's diabetes," the doctor says. "I think his adrenal cortex isn't working right."
Which adrenal cortex hormone is related to blood pressure and salt levels? How is it related to them? Do you think this boy has too much of that hormone, or too little?
ALDOSTERONE controls the reabsorption of Na^+ and water in the kidneys, by activating the Na^+/K^+ ATPase.
The boy has too little ALDOSTERONE, so he isn't running the Na^+/K^+ ATPase in his kidneys. As a result, he's losing Na^+ and water in his urine, a condition called 'salt wasting.' This is evidenced by his high urine volume, low blood pressure, and salt craving.

Which adrenal cortex hormone is related to blood glucose levels? How is it related to them? Do you think this boy has too much of that hormone, or too little?
CORTISOL causes cells to release glucose into the blood. This is a key part of your response to stress, as it provides a fast energy source for your body.
The boy's blood glucose is low, so he probably has lowCORTISOL as well. This might explain his liking for sweet snacks as well (but doesn't everybody like those?)

The doctor has ordered blood tests for [K^+], ACTH, andCORTISOL. Why are these tests relevant, and what do you expect their values to be? (high, normal, or low)
The doctor is testingCORTISOL levels to see whether the hypothesis that the adrenal cortex isn't working is correct. If it is,CORTISOL levels will be low. But the doctor also wants to know whether the anterior pituitary is working correctly, which will be revealed by the ACTH test. Finally, the doctor tests [K^+] levels because it is controlled by the Na^+/K^+ ATPase in the kidneys. If the boy has low ALDOSTERONE and isn't running that pump, it will not be moving K^+ into the urine and blood K^+ levels could build up – which could alter nerve and muscle firing and lead to cardiac arrest.

The tests show thatCORTISOL levels are low, but ACTH is high. Does this indicate that there is a problem with the boy's anterior pituitary as well as his adrenal cortex?
This is normal! IfCORTISOL is low, the hypothalamus and anterior pituitary will detect that and begin to release the hormones that stimulateCORTISOL production. ACTH will increase.

Key for Parathyroid Function and Parathyroid Disorders

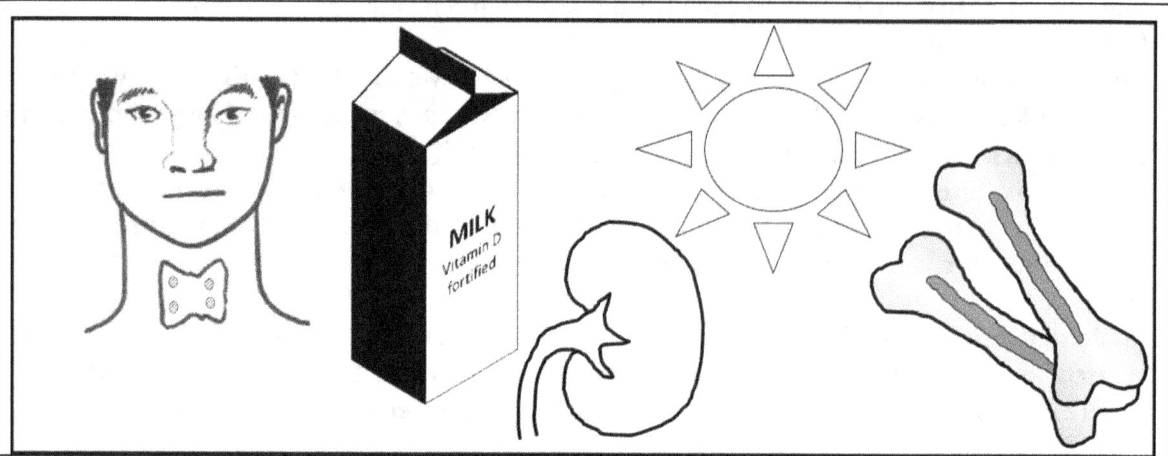

Here are your parathyroids, shown in green. They are attached to the back of your thyroid.

When blood <u>calcium</u> levels are too low, they secrete <u>PARATHYROID HORMONE</u>.

This hormone helps you bring blood <u>calcium</u> levels back up to normal. It helps you absorb <u>calcium</u> from your diet.

It also helps you reabsorb it from your <u>urine</u> into your <u>blood</u>.

When blood <u>calcium</u> levels return to normal, the parathyroids will <u>stop</u> secreting <u>PARATHYROID HORMONE</u>.

<u>Vitamin D3</u> is also needed for you to <u>absorb</u> calcium.

You can make this compound when your skin is exposed to <u>UV light</u>, or you can get it from your diet. You can only absorb it from your diet if you are able to digest <u>fats</u>.

Whether you made or absorbed it, you have to activate it in your <u>kidneys</u> before it can help you with calcium balance.

When they first begin secreting <u>PARATHYROID HORMONE</u>, the parathyroids stimulate <u>osteoblasts</u>. The <u>calcium</u> you're absorbing will be deposited in your <u>bones</u>. Two other factors that will help you deposit calcium in your bones are <u>ESTROGEN</u> and <u>load-bearing exercise</u>.

If <u>PARATHYROID HORMONE</u> levels remain high for too long, though, the <u>osteoclasts</u> will be stimulated and they will start to release <u>calcium</u> from your <u>bones</u> into the blood.

Bone image from Pixabay, https://pixabay.com/en/bone-dog-skeleton-157272/ : public domain

Key for Kidney Function and Renal Disorders

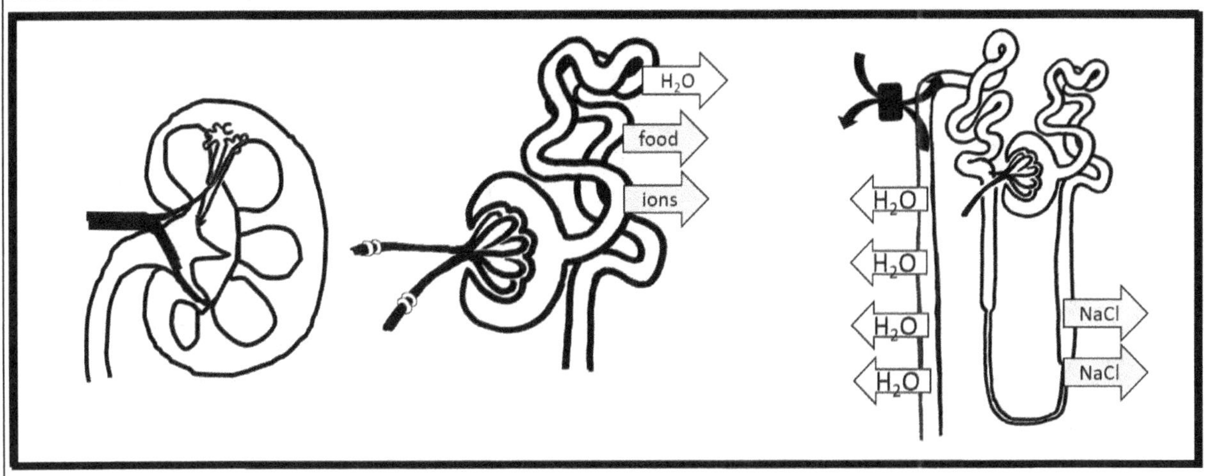

Here's one of your kidneys, filtering your blood. The blood enters through the <u>renal artery</u>, which branches until it forms many <u>afferent arterioles</u>. Each of these sends blood into a tiny capillary bed called a <u>glomerulus</u>. After it's been filtered, the blood leaves through the <u>efferent arterioles</u>, which return it to the <u>renal vein</u>.

The total amount of blood filtered in all these capillary beds is called the <u>glomerular filtration rate</u>, and it is about 125 mL/ minute.
The outer layer of the kidneys, containing the filters, is called the <u>cortex</u>. The salty inner layer is the <u>medulla</u>.

Here's one of your renal tubules, or <u>nephrons</u>. Each of these gets ultrafiltrate from its own <u>glomerulus</u>. At the other end, the tubule empties into the renal <u>calyx</u>, which sends it down the <u>ureter</u> to the <u>bladder</u>.

The first part of the tubule, <u>Bowman's capsule</u>, collects the ultrafiltrate. Everything in the blood except <u>cells</u>, <u>proteins</u> and <u>lipids</u> can pass through the filter into the ultrafiltrate, but about <u>70</u>% of the solutes and water are reabsorbed in the <u>proximal convoluted tubule</u>.
More Na$^+$ and water can also be reabsorbed in the <u>DCT</u>, but only if the hormone <u>ALDOSTERONE</u> has turned on the <u>Na$^+$/K$^+$ATPase</u>. This ATPase is also used to remove <u>K$^+$</u> from the blood.

When ultrafiltrate passes through the Loop of <u>Henle</u>, Na$^+$ and Cl- are reabsorbed into the renal <u>medulla</u>, making it <u>hypertonic</u>. This is important because later, when ultrafiltrate passes down the <u>collecting duct</u> through this area, water can be <u>reabsorbed</u> from the urine into the medulla by osmosis. That will only happen if the hormone <u>ADH</u> has made the duct permeable to water.
The kidneys respond to low blood flow in the <u>afferent</u> arteriole by secreting <u>renin</u>, which activates the <u>RAA</u> system and increases <u>ALDOSTERONE</u> secretion so that the <u>Na$^+$/K$^+$</u> ATPase will reabsorb <u>Na$^+$ and H2O</u>, making blood volume go <u>up</u>.
If blood O$_2$ levels are low, the kidneys secrete <u>ERYTHROPOIETIN</u> to stimulate RBC production in the bone marrow. And the kidneys activate <u>vitamin D3</u>, which is needed for you to absorb <u>calcium</u> from your diet.

Key for Motor Function and Motor Disorders

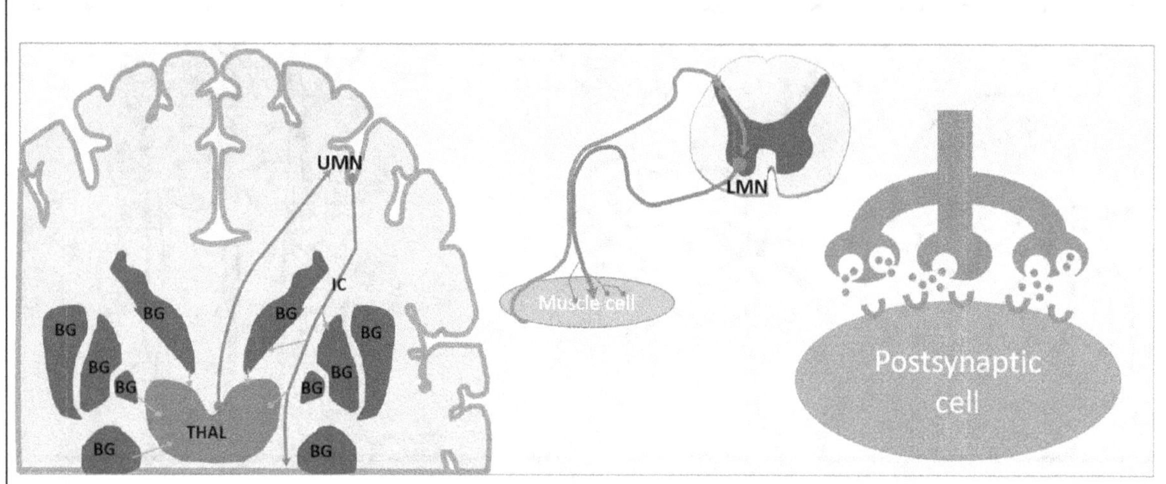

Here are the <u>upper motor</u> neurons in your <u>cerebral cortex</u>. Each of them controls a specific part of your body. To do that, they have to send their axons down through the <u>internal capsule</u> to the <u>white</u> matter of the <u>spinal cord</u>.

The motor impulses are also sent to the <u>thalamus</u> and <u>basal ganglia</u>, which control whether the movement can occur. The neurotransmitter <u>GABA</u> prevents unplanned movements, while the neurotransmitter <u>dopamine</u> reinforces planned movements.

The axons synapse with <u>lower motor neurons</u> living in the <u>gray matter</u> of the spinal cord.

These neurons interact with each other to run spinal reflexes like the <u>Babinski</u> reflex, <u>muscle tone</u>, and <u>patterned gait generation</u>. These don't need your brain to work, but your upper motor neurons can modulate them.

Axons from the <u>lower motor neurons</u> leave the spine as the <u>ventral</u> roots of the <u>spinal</u> nerves.

Axons from the <u>lower motor neurons</u> make up the <u>motor</u> nerves, which carry the signal to the muscles. To make the signal move fast enough, these nerves are coated with <u>myelin</u>. The muscle cells controlled by each neuron are its <u>motor unit</u>. They will all contract together when that neuron fires.

The neuron makes them fire by releasing <u>acetylcholine</u>, which lands on <u>nicotinic</u> receptors on the muscle cells and makes them <u>depolarize</u>. The <u>acetylcholine</u> is then removed by the enzyme <u>acetylcholinesterase</u>, and the muscle can relax.

Mrs. B is 72 years old and complains of leg weakness. She says it's been getting progressively worse. The doctor and the Physician Assistant are discussing her case and they've come up with a list of diseases to investigate and try to rule out.
How could each of these diseases have caused her leg weakness?
Stroke is when a clot or a broken blood vessel cuts off the oxygen supply to cells in the cerebral cortex, killing or injuring them.
A stroke that cut off blood flow to cells in Mrs. B's motor cortex could damage the cells that send motor impulses to her legs. There wouldn't be anything wrong with her legs, but she just wouldn't be able to send them instructions to move.

Parkinson's Disease is when the basal ganglia lose their ability to make dopamine.
Without dopamine, the basal ganglia cannot tell the thalamus to reinforce a planned motion. The person's movements become smaller and require more effort – and they may eventually not be able to move when they want to.

Multiple sclerosis is when axons in the central nervous system begin to lose their myelin coating.
Myelin makes the impulses run down the axons more quickly. If some of the axons have lost their myelin, then some of the impulses will move more slowly than others. Impulses won't reach the muscles in a normal coordinated fashion.

Myasthenia gravis is a disorder that destroys nicotinic receptors on the skeletal muscle cells.
Muscle cells fire when acetylcholine released from motor neurons attaches to the nicotinic receptors. As those receptors are destroyed, the muscle cells become less able to respond to the motor nerves.

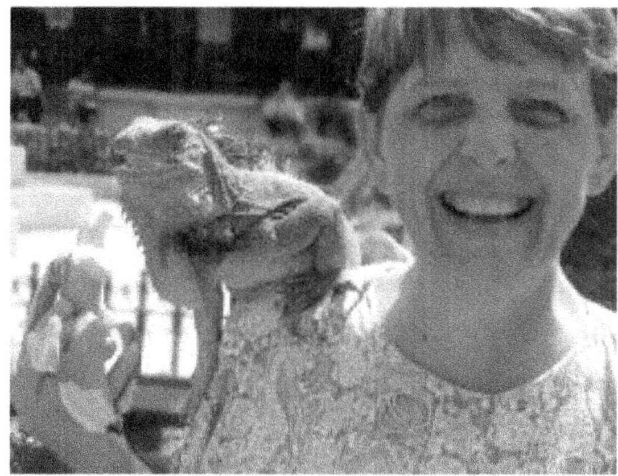

Hello, and pleased to meet you!

I've been teaching A&P and Pathophysiology to nursing majors for over 30 years, and have also taught Graduate Pathophysiology in the MSN program.

It's been one of the most worthwhile experiences in my life to study, organize, and teach this endlessly fascinating material. Even more rewarding is my interaction with students who are interested and informed about the area, and whose questions constantly push me to refine my knowledge and think more rigorously about its clinical applications.

Working with nursing students and nurses is an honor and a delight. My professional goal, and the goal of this book, is to make it easier for you to learn the material that will help you save lives.

I hope it helps make Patho a fun application of principles, rather than a mere task of memorizing.

You can find more resources, and about my other career as a writer, at my website: www.raosyth.com or www.patbowne.com.

Enjoy!